IT'S NOT YOU, IT'S YOUR HORMONES

The essential guide for women over 40 to fight fat, fatigue and hormone havoc

by Nicki Williams

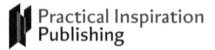

Practical Inspiration Publishing

PRAISE FOR *IT'S NOT YOU, IT'S YOUR HORMONES*

In my line of work I meet a lot of women suffering from 'tired all the time' and other more specific hormone issues. This book is a must-have for every woman over 40! Hormone health is integral to every aspect of a woman's life, from increasing your confidence to having the energy to achieve what you want in life. Nicki's mission is to fully empower women with the knowledge and tools they need so that they don't have to suffer in silence, and can reach their full potential.

Dr Joanna Martin, founder of One of many

As a mother of three who works with women every day, I know for certain that hormones are the invisible key to feeling healthy and happy. Nicki Williams has dedicated her life's work to empowering women to understand and work with their bodies so they can stay their most beautiful, powerful and fulfilled. I'm an absolutely huge fan of her philosophy and her work in the world – it is so needed! This book will give you the tools and support you need to feel and look amazing for years to come.

Katharine Dever, Intuitive Business Consultant, Inspirational Speaker and Author

If your hormones are misbehaving, leaving you tired, wired, overweight and bloated (to name just a few undesirable symptoms) then you need this book! Nicki tells you everything you need to know about your hormones in a simple, authoritative and entertaining way. Follow her expert advice to reclaim your health, vitality and the body you deserve.

Linda Munster, Nutritionist and Author of *No Caffeine Required*

Too many women believe that there are only two choices for dealing with menopause symptoms: you either take hormone replacement therapy or you put up with it. Wrong! In this book Nicki Williams sets out clearly the connection between diet and the commonly experienced symptoms. More importantly she provides simple adjustments you can make to your diet and lifestyle to achieve significant beneficial results. A must-read for women over 40.

Pat Duckworth, Midlife Therapist and Award-Winning Author of *Hot Women, Cool Solutions*

Nicki Williams approaches the thorny subject of hormones in a practical, no-nonsense and pragmatic way in this brilliant new book. With Nicki's wonderfully clean and clear narrative, you are in no doubt that hormones have a huge role to play in who we are, how we feel and how we react to life. You couldn't wish for a better, more professional and experienced guide to take you to a brilliant, healthy, supercharged future beyond the despair you might be feeling now.

Kate Cook, International Speaker, Author, Nutritionist and Wellness Expert

A MUST READ for all women suffering from mood swings, weight gain, fatigue or brain fog.

Dr Wendy Denning, Integrated Private GP and co-author of *Diet Doctors: Inside and Out*

Hormone imbalances can cause untold misery, yet it really doesn't have to be that way. Nicki's book demystifies what can be a daunting subject and her holistic approach will empower women to take control of their hormones and their health.

Glen Matten, Nutritional Medicine Consultant and author of *The Sirtfood Diet*

ABOUT THE AUTHOR

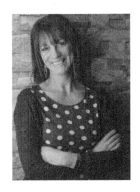 Nicki Williams, DipION, mBANT, CNHC, is a qualified Nutritional Therapist, speaker and founder of Happy Hormones for Life, helping women to rebalance their hormones, reclaim their health and feel better than ever.

After failing to find any medical help for her symptoms of exhaustion, weight gain and hormone issues in her early 40s, she discovered it was her hormones that were at fault and that she could turn things around using diet, lifestyle and natural supplements.

She went on to qualify as a Nutritional Therapist at the renowned Institute of Optimum Nutrition (ION), making hormones her speciality. She and her team now help women all over the world with online programmes, workshops and corporate, individual and group coaching.

In their one-to-one work, they use state-of-the-art comprehensive hormone (and other) testing and Functional Medicine principles to identify the root cause of any imbalance and provide fully personalized programmes for faster targeted results.

www.happyhormonesforlife.com

www.facebook.com/happyhormonesforlife

@nickijwilliams

@happyhormonesforlife

Linked in. www.linkedin.com/in/williamsnicki

TABLE OF CONTENTS

INTRODUCTION

'What the hell has happened to me since I hit 40?' If you are asking yourself that question you have picked up the right book.

You may be suffering and feeling lost, or you may just have started noticing some changes. Either way, you're probably looking for some answers and not getting very far.

If this is you, then you're one of the 80% of women that are thought to suffer from various symptoms between the ages of 35 and 60, yet there is very little awareness and support available. According to a UK survey of over 3000 women aged over 40, conducted by Nuffield Health in 2014, many suffered anxiety, depression, had to take regular time off work and two thirds of them said there was not enough help available. And over half of them failed to recognize that any of their symptoms were due to hormone imbalances, citing they were either too young or too old.

You might assume or have been told that you are 'just getting older', or you may have been to your doctor who offered you antidepressants or HRT. Or you may have tried the latest diet and exercise programmes or miracle supplements that promise to 'fix' you.

None of these 'solutions' have worked? That's because none of them are addressing the true cause of your symptoms: your hormones!

Whether you are in perimenopause (the years running up to menopause), or you are post-menopausal, hormone imbalances can cause havoc.

Every woman has a different experience, but common symptoms are fatigue, stubborn weight gain (especially around the middle), mood swings, brain fog, insomnia, hot flushes, PMS and more! Or you may just feel like something is off, that you've lost your mojo.

Your hormones control your energy, mood, sex drive, stress response and fat stores, amongst other critical functions. As you age your hormones decline and fluctuate at varying rates, upsetting the delicate balance and causing all sorts of unwanted side effects.

When they are nice and balanced, you can expect to feel full of energy, to be in control of your weight, to have balanced moods throughout the month, a clear, focused mind, glowing skin, restorative sleep and a calm, happy outlook.

Sounds impossible? I thought that too. But it's not. Your symptoms can be alleviated by some simple changes to your diet and lifestyle.

By looking after your hormones and giving them what they need, they will look after you in return. This book will show you how to give your hormones the TLC they need so that you can feel great again, sail through menopause and come out stronger and healthier than before.

My story

These days, I am a qualified nutritionist and hormone specialist, but I wasn't always interested in healthy food and hormones! In fact, far from it. I was the chubby kid at school. I loved food, especially CAKE – any kind, any flavour.

Seven stone at age seven, my mum sent me to kiddies' Weightwatchers and there began my introduction to a life of yo-yo dieting. I don't know if there was any deep-seated psychological reason for my love of food. I had a very loving family. But we moved a lot, and maybe it was my way of feeling better about always being the new kid in school.

Cake is still my weakness today. I can resist pretty much anything, but put me in front of a gooey chocolate cake and I go back to being the fat new kid at school.

In my teens I got tall so the weight redistributed a bit. I became more obsessed with dieting though, and remember taking an apple to school for lunch. I would 'treat' myself to some low fat cottage cheese on a cracker when I got home and lived on Diet Coke to get my sweet fix.

At university, I binged on alcohol and pizza then would starve for a few days to rebalance. I knew it wasn't healthy but it meant I could be 'normal' for at least some of the time.

In my 20s I carried on partying, working in an office and counting down to the weekend – getting drunk and eating rubbish. I couldn't cook (even though I had been brought up on amazing home-cooked food!) and relied on packet food and frozen TV dinners.

In my 30s I got married and had kids. But despite having little ones learning my unhealthy ways, I wasn't about to change my eating (and drinking) habits any time soon. I was still getting away with it.

But when I hit 40 everything changed. I suddenly couldn't get away with it any longer. I couldn't lose my muffin top, despite every fad diet going, my weekend hangovers were getting worse, I felt achy and cold, and frankly exhausted.

I had a busy job, two gorgeous but demanding children and all the other things women have to juggle: family, friends, school runs, exercise, food shopping, cooking, cleaning, getting my hair/nails/legs done and somehow finding time to relax (which never happened!).

I didn't like myself at all. I was grumpy with my husband, snappy with the kids and generally angry with everyone else. I felt like I had lost myself, and was starting to worry I was going to lose everyone else too.

Life felt like a never-ending treadmill. But I didn't have the energy to do anything about it.

Until a cold January evening in 2007. I had been at work, come home, fed the kids and was standing at the kitchen sink wondering how on earth I was going to complete a report for my boss for the next day when I could hardly keep my eyes open. My daughter was seven at the time, she came running in to show me a picture she had drawn at school of a giraffe (she knew it was my favourite animal). 'Mummy, Mummy, look at what I did today!' I spun around and shouted, 'Not now, Sasha!' Her little face crumpled and she growled, 'Why are you always so grumpy, Mummy?' and flounced out of the room.

That was my trigger. It was like a stab in the back. I had become a 'Grumpy Mum', something I never wanted to be. I wanted to be a fun mum! I decided enough was enough. Something had to be done.

I went to my doctor. I reeled off all my symptoms, taking up most of the 10-minute appointment we had. He patiently sat at his computer typing. When I had finished my rant, he handed me a prescription. I looked down at the word. 'Prozac?' I said, 'But Doctor, I'm not depressed' and he said, 'It'll make you feel better' as he ushered me out.

I sat in the car outside the surgery and burst into tears. Maybe I was depressed? But I knew deep down that this wasn't the answer for me.

And that's when I rang my dad. He's also a doctor. You might think why on earth didn't I just ask him for advice? Well, I come from a long line of doctors – going back decades. I had the grades to study medicine but I rebelled against tradition and studied languages. I had never really taken any notice of my dad's advice, despite him turning away from traditional 'drug based' medicine to a more natural approach. He had suffered from Chronic Fatigue Syndrome (or ME) for years and cured himself using food, supplements and lifestyle changes. I guess now I was finally ready to listen.

The conversation went a bit like this:
Me: 'Hi Dad, I really need your help. My doctor thinks I'm depressed, and maybe I am! My life's a mess – I'm exhausted, overweight, I can't think straight and my kids hate me!'
Dad: 'Ah don't worry Nick, I see this in my clinic all the time – it'll be your hormones. You're in peri-menopause.'
Me: '*Peri-what*? Did you just say menopause? I'm only 42. What do you mean?'
Dad: 'Hormones start to change after 35; that's when you start 'peri' menopause. You're just feeling the effects now. Don't worry we'll get you tested…'

I was pretty shocked about this news! I knew nothing about my hormones. I just thought they were about puberty, pregnancy, PMS and menopause in your fifties! I didn't know about the peri-menopause and the symptoms that came with it.

And fair enough, he was right. We discovered I had several hormone imbalances, including adrenal fatigue, low thyroid and low progesterone. I had been overstressed for years juggling a family and career, and was in the midst of perimenopause! Thank goodness it wasn't all in my head. There was actually something physical going on, which was a huge relief.

He recommended some simple changes to my diet and lifestyle, and started me on some targeted supplements. I was amazed that I started to feel better really quickly. I lost the weight I had been clinging on to, I had loads more energy, felt much happier and balanced. This was good stuff.

And the BEST thing? I didn't have to give up my favourite things – coffee, chocolate and wine!

I was so impressed by my results that I made the momentous decision to go back to college and learn about nutrition properly.

After four years of lectures, seminars, assignments and clinical practice, I learnt how to properly look after my hormones with the right foods, supplements and lifestyle choices. I created a simple four-step system that I use myself and with my clients to get hormones rebalanced. And the great news is that you don't have to do it the hard way, just read this book and you'll learn how to do it for yourself.

I am now sailing through perimenopause with relative ease. I'm certainly not perfect – I still love my wine, coffee and chocolate. But I have found a system that works for me and keeps me sane. As I write this, I am 49 and feel better than I have in years. I am very rarely ill, have loads of energy and am maintaining a healthy weight (plus/minus the odd few pounds after holidays!).

And I'm on a MISSION! To educate and empower other women to regain control of their hormones so that they don't have to suffer needlessly.

You don't have to just accept that you're getting older (as many doctors will tell you). You don't have to be a slave to your hormones, at any age.

Because women are at the hub of their families, workplaces and communities and when they are at their best everyone around them benefits. The ripple effect can be enormous. I'd even like to think it might save a few marriages!

My dad is still my inspiration (and medical encyclopaedia) – he never judged my errant ways or put pressure on me to follow in his footsteps, but I definitely felt his pride when I told him I wanted to study nutrition. Maybe I was always destined to follow the doctor genes in the family, but by stubbornly doing it my way instead.

So I have written this book to share the exact process that I use on myself and my clients to achieve hormonal harmony, allowing the body to release excess weight, restore youthful energy levels, balance moods and clear out the brain fog. Oh and let you sail through the menopause and beyond, when it's your time.

By understanding what happens to your hormones as you get older, why hormone imbalances can make you feel tired, fat, moody, stressed and unsexy, and what you can do about it naturally, you'll be able to turn things around very quickly.

I will concentrate on the four main hormonal imbalances that are responsible for many of the health issues you might be facing in your 40s, and which respond really well to some TLC in the form of good nutrition and lifestyle choices.

The choices you make about what you eat and how you live your life have a profound impact on your hormones. And it's so much easier than you might think.

All that I ask from you is that you make the commitment to yourself – either take the information in this book and follow it yourself or find an expert to guide you.

This book is not a miracle cure and there is never a 'one-size-fits-all' solution. It's always best to work with a qualified practitioner who can test your hormone levels and give you a personalized programme. However, there are generic dietary and lifestyle shifts that can make a huge difference. And once you start making small changes, you will start to notice big improvements.

The most important thing is to get started. Everything is easier once you make the commitment.

Enjoy the journey!

A QUICK GUIDE TO GETTING THE MOST OUT OF THIS BOOK

The workbook

I have created a workbook to accompany this book, which will help you answer the questions raised and make your own personal plan. You can download it at www.happyhormonesforlife.com/book. It is electronic, so you don't need to print it off, but once you have completed it, there is an option to save as a PDF and you can print it from there.

What we're going to cover

Part 1 is your hormone education. To understand is to control! Once you understand what's happening in your own body, you are so much more in control of it. Chapter 1 is a bit of background on hormones and the way they control how we look, feel, think and behave. If you're wondering if you even have a hormone imbalance, you can find out the likely culprit by taking the quiz in Chapter 2. Chapter 3 is where you get intimate with your Feisty 4, the main hormones that you need to know about after 40.

In Part 2, you'll learn why your hormones are in desperate need of your help. Chapter 4 covers the big four influences – the things you do on a daily basis, the choices you make and the thoughts you have, and how they affect your hormones and how they work. If you know how your choices affect your life, then you have the power to change things. In Chapter 5 we look at why you should ditch the diet and low fat mantra we have all been following for too long. And in Chapter 6, I'll explain how your gut and liver are connected to your hormones and why it's important to look after them.

Part 3 is where we put it all together! In Chapter 7, I take you through the simple four-step process that I have used on myself and on my clients to regain control of the Feisty 4 hormones, and lose that stubborn weight, regain energy, balance moods and clear the brain fog. In Chapter 8, we look at how you need to get your head in the right place before you even start with the body, and in Chapter 9 it's all about maintenance – how to keep the good habits going for life.

In Part 4 you can find out how to step it up a gear; how to get tested for hormone imbalances, what supplements are best for women over 40, and the low-down on HRT and BHRT.

Journaling

I'm a big fan of writing stuff down. If I'm doing a new course or reading a new book, I love to buy myself a lovely notebook to write all my new learnings in. I've provided you with a workbook for the main questions, but I really encourage you to make your own notes where you can as you go through the book. There will be parts that resonate with you more than others, so scribble them down. I really love doing a food journal too. Writing down everything you eat helps with awareness of your habits, but it also helps to add in any symptoms you experience when you eat certain foods, particularly helpful if you suspect you may have any food intolerances. Food diaries have also been shown to help with weight loss (even if you make no additional changes!).

Resources

Towards the end of the book I have included a selection of my favourite resources to help you put the principles of the book into practice, including some of my favourite hormone-balancing recipes, guides and further reading. They are available to download and print out at www.happyhormonesforlife.com/book.

Disclaimer

The information presented in this book is for informational purposes only and is not intended as a substitute for advice from your physician or doctor or other health care professional.

You should consult with a physician, doctor or health care professional before undertaking any diet, exercise or supplement programme, before taking any medication or nutritional supplement, or if you have or suspect you might have a health problem.

The author and publishers cannot be held responsible for any errors and omissions that may be found in the text or any actions that may be taken by a reader as a result of any reliance on the information contained in the text, which is taken entirely at the reader's own risk.

PART 1

HERE'S THE THING ABOUT HORMONES

CHAPTER 1

HORMONES 101 – WHAT ARE THEY AND WHY DO THEY AFFECT US SO MUCH?

Personally I think hormones are fascinating, but I get it if you don't share my passion! The thing is, if you're over 40, you should probably take a bit of interest because they are going to take you on a journey, and if you want it to be a fun ride then you're going to want to be in the driving seat and not an unwilling passenger.

Women just don't get the information they need about what happens to their own bodies. And they certainly don't get enough help from the people who are supposed to know about these things.

The only thing to do is to take responsibility for your own health. Knowledge is definitely power, and the more you know the more you will be in control of your journey.

What are hormones?

Hormones get a bad rap generally. They are blamed for everything from teenage angst to crazy PMS. But if you ask anyone to name their hormones, they might tell you about oestrogen and testosterone. Some might even remember that cortisol is your 'stress hormone', or serotonin your 'happy hormone'. The thyroid might get a mention, but did you know that insulin is one of your most important hormones? Or that you have special hormones that control your appetite?

If, like me, you thought hormone issues were just about PMS, pregnancy and menopause, you are not alone. Many of us, including a lot of doctors, are unaware of the extent to which hormones rule our lives.

From conception to birth and beyond, hormones are the driving force behind every biological and physiological process in the body. Even if you have heard of the main hormones, you might not know what they do and why you need them. You don't need to know this (and if this doesn't interest you, you can check your hormone imbalance in Chapter 2, then skip straight to the relevant chapter), but if you are interested in improving your health, it's worth getting to know your hormones a little better. That way you will know how to make them happy so that they will look after you.

These mysterious chemicals flow through every part of our body and pretty much control everything we do. They change children into adults, help those adults make children, and have a huge influence over how you feel, think, eat, move, metabolize, digest, sleep and function.

There are over 100 identified hormones in the body. They are made in the endocrine glands and travel around in your blood, billions of units at a time, to practically every cell of your body. From the Greek word 'hormon', meaning to set in motion or excite, hormones are chemical messengers that tell the body's cells what to do.

Hormones are everywhere, trying to look after your body as best they can. Every hormone has a job to do, some are general and act on nearly every cell (like the thyroid), others have very specific roles (like aldosterone, which acts on the kidney to retain water). Here's a selection of what they do on a daily basis. They:

- control your heartbeat, breathing and blood pressure

- allow you to sleep at night and wake in the morning
- control your hunger, metabolism and growth
- determine your masculine and feminine traits, and reproductive function
- build bone, repair skin and muscle
- regulate fat stores
- control your energy levels, mood and stress resistance
- regulate brain activity – thinking, memory, focus, mood
- control blood sugar levels and stimulate your immune system
- lessen pain and make you happy

All in all, you can't live without them! And when they are all working optimally, you are going to be generally healthy (aside from non-hormonal conditions). However, in modern life and as you age, there are several challenges that hormones face that can tip them out of balance and cause symptoms in many different areas of the body. And if not addressed, this can lead to more serious conditions, such as diabetes, heart disease, obesity, dementia, osteoporosis and cancer.

The top 10 hormone symptoms

So many women I speak to don't realize that their symptoms are due to hormone imbalances. That's because hormone changes don't happen overnight, they creep up on you very gradually so that you just get used to the extra tiredness, or the brain fog, and it's often a trigger or event that makes you sit up and take notice (mine was my daughter telling me I was a grumpy mum!).

You might have noticed your friends going through similar things too, so it's easy to assume that this is a normal part of ageing and it's just what happens. And often that's what your doctor will tell you too. 'Just get on with it, you're getting older!'

And menopause happens in your 50s, right? Anyway, you're not having hot flushes, so it can't be that, can it? While it's true that your periods finally stop in your 50s (mostly), the perimenopause transition can last up to 17 years! And you don't need to be having hot flushes to be going through it…

So if you're wondering if your symptoms could be hormonal, here are the top 10 common complaints you might not realize can be hormone issues.

1. **Weight gain.** You've got stubborn fat that has crept up on you over the years, or a spare tyre that's impossible to shift no matter what diet or exercise you try. You have gone up a clothes size or two and are so frustrated you can't wear those gorgeous clothes that you used to. Your metabolism is getting slower, yet you're always hungry! You've tried the 'eat less, move more' approach, and it just makes you miserable. And you're still overweight. **Time to sort out your hormones!**

   Potential imbalances: cortisol, thyroid, insulin, oestrogen.

2. **Tired All The Time.** 'TATT' is by far the most common complaint from women I see in my clinic. You just don't have the energy you used to have. It's a struggle to get through the day without feeling drowsy or sluggish (especially mid afternoon and late evening). You think it's just what happens when you get older and, after all, you have a really busy life. But it's not normal to be tired all the time. **Get your hormones in balance** and you'll get your energy back.

   Potential imbalances: cortisol, thyroid, insulin.

3. **Stressed out.** You are the Queen of multi-tasking! Always rushing from one thing to the next, juggling many responsibilities at once, and feeling overwhelmed most of

the time. 'Me time' is nowhere near your to-do list, let alone on it. You're not sleeping great, getting irritated easily, feeling wired, tired and just about holding it together. You probably feel guilty relaxing, or try to slow down but just can't switch off. If you feel like you're on a never-ending hamster wheel, you need to **start looking after your hormones**.

Potential imbalance: cortisol.

4. **Mood swings.** You may have had mood swings when you were younger, but these days they are more extreme. You have a lot more down days where you lack motivation and drive. You have little patience and often snap at those closest to you (let alone that maniac who just tried to cut you up!). **This isn't YOU; it's your HORMONES.**

Potential imbalances: cortisol, thyroid, insulin, oestrogen.

5. **Memory loss and brain fog.** You used to be such a sharp cookie. You can feel it slipping. You can't concentrate for long any more, have trouble solving problems and making key decisions. You walk into a room and forget what you wanted. You forget names and what you were going to say in the middle of your ....

It can be scary – we've all seen films like *Still Alice*. Or we might know or be caring for elderly relatives with Alzheimer's or dementia. But more often than not, it's common-or-garden BRAIN FOG that's driving us crazy. And it's **hormones at the root of it.**

Potential imbalances: cortisol, thyroid, insulin, oestrogen.

6. **PMS and period chaos.** You thought PMS was over for you now you are heading towards menopause, but it seems to be worse! Your periods are too heavy (or too light), too frequent (or infrequent), and you might have PMS symptoms for

most of the month. This one is obviously **hormonal**, but you might not understand why it's getting so much worse.

Potential imbalances: cortisol, thyroid, insulin, oestrogen.

7. **Low sex drive.** So you used to get excited about sex with your partner, now it's the last thing on your mind! Sometimes you're too exhausted, other times you just can't get in the mood. What happened to the sex kitten you used to be? Sex isn't compulsory as you get older, and many women are happy not to worry about it anymore. But sex is really good for you and if you still want to have a good sex life, you may just need to **balance your hormones**.

Potential imbalances: cortisol, thyroid, oestrogen, testosterone.

8. **Anxiety.** Were you ever this worried about the small things? You seem to worry about everything these days: the kids, work, money, relationships, friends, the future. You can get really emotional about the tiniest thing. Suddenly crying for no apparent reason? **It's your hormones!**

Potential imbalances: cortisol, thyroid, oestrogen.

9. **Hair, skin and nails**. You didn't use to worry about your hair, skin or nails. They were just fine. Now, your hair's thinning on your head but growing in other places, your nails are brittle or cracked, and your skin is dry, itchy, puffy and you're getting deep wrinkles. And you're having breakouts like a teenager! Is this part of getting older, or **is it your hormones?**

Potential imbalances: cortisol, thyroid, oestrogen.

10. **Digestive issues.** Your digestion problems are getting worse. You're suffering from constipation, diarrhoea, indigestion,

bloating or gas. And you've got food intolerances you never used to have. That's often because **your hormones and your digestion are intimately connected.**

Potential imbalances: cortisol, thyroid.

And of course I'm not going to leave out the most obvious menopause symptom…

Hot Flushes and Night Sweats

As oestrogen is swinging from high to low during perimenopause, these fluctuations can cause hot flushes (or flashes) and increased sweating at night. Scientists aren't completely sure of the mechanism, but it's thought that oestrogen has an important role in thermoregulation. So when oestrogen dips, your temperature control can go haywire and you can find yourself burning up like a furnace, dripping with sweat and wanting to dive into a freezer for some relief!

Potential imbalances: cortisol, oestrogen.

So if you recognize any of these common complaints, you are reading the right book! Jump to Chapter 2 and take the quiz to see which of your hormones may be playing up.

PCOS, endometriosis and fibroids

While natural ageing is certainly a factor in many hormone-related symptoms, there are some more chronic hormone-driven conditions that can occur at any age. This book isn't aimed at these specific hormone conditions, as there are many complex factors involved and each case is unique and needs a personalized approach. However, I have selected a few common conditions that are related to hormone imbalances and respond really well to the natural protocols that I talk about in Part 3.

PCOS – Polycystic Ovarian Syndrome

PCOS is a very common condition describing a set of symptoms that can include missing or delayed ovulation, excess androgens (acne, facial hair, hair loss), weight gain, insulin resistance and infertility. As well as these distressing symptoms, long-term PCOS can increase your risk of diabetes, heart disease and cancer.

You may have had an ultrasound to see if you have multiple cysts on your ovaries. These are caused by undeveloped follicles that have not properly matured enough at the time of ovulation to allow the egg to break through. Although PCOS is named after these cysts, it's actually not a prerequisite for a diagnosis of PCOS, and equally you may have cysts showing up but not have PCOS as your ovaries change every month. Either way, it's important to get some tests done to confirm that you actually have PCOS.

The many factors behind PCOS

Insulin resistance

A diet high in carbs and sugar over the long term can cause the insulin receptors on your cells to shut down (see more on insulin in Chapter 3), allowing higher levels of insulin to be released by the pancreas. Too much insulin can:

- interfere with ovulation
- stimulate your ovaries to make androgens instead of oestrogen
- trigger your pituitary gland to make too much LH (luteinizing hormone)
- reduce SHBG (sex hormone binding globulin), which increases free testosterone

Weight gain
Fat tissue produces an enzyme called aromatase, which increases androgens, so the more overweight you are, the more testosterone and androgens you are likely to be producing.

Stress
Excess stress hormones (see more on cortisol in Chapter 3) can interfere with ovulation by suppressing oestrogen and progesterone. Cortisol also increases insulin (see earlier).

Inflammation (especially in your gut!)
Inflammation damages your hormone receptors and suppresses ovulation. If you have any gut imbalance (see Chapter 6) you will have inflammation happening, so sorting out your digestive health may help with your PCOS.

Low thyroid hormones
If you don't have enough active thyroid hormone, your ovaries might not have the energy they need to ovulate. Low thyroid also stimulates the production of prolactin (a hormone produced during breastfeeding that stops you getting pregnant).

Nutrient deficiencies
Specific nutrients are needed by your ovaries to function properly (releasing that follicle at ovulation). These include iodine, selenium, vitamin D and zinc, and deficiencies can interfere with ovulation.

The good news is that if you adopt the principles in Chapter 7 and work with a qualified health practitioner, symptoms of PCOS can be significantly improved.

Endometriosis

Endometriosis is a painful condition whereby parts of your uterine tissue grow outside of your uterus (like having a period from the wrong place). These endometrial lesions can grow anywhere in your body, but are most common in the ovaries, fallopian tubes, bowel and bladder. They are sensitive to oestrogen so they bleed with your menstrual cycle causing heavy periods, pain and inflammation. It's thought to be caused by an overactive immune response to your own tissue – an autoimmune disease more than a hormonal condition, but more research is needed.

As the condition is worsened by high oestrogen levels, a hormone-balancing diet and lifestyle (especially removing dairy and gluten), supporting the liver and reducing environmental oestrogen exposure can all help to relieve symptoms until post-menopause, when the condition naturally dissipates.

Fibroids

Fibroids are common during perimenopause when progesterone levels decline and leave oestrogen dominant. They are smooth muscle tumours found inside and outside the uterine wall, and can cause heavy and painful periods, and interfere with fertility.

As oestrogen levels decline after menopause, fibroids do generally disappear. But while you are waiting, you can really improve your symptoms by adopting the principles in Chapter 7.

The key hormones you need to know about

Science alert!!
If it's a while since you did biology at school (or like me you were more interested in the boy in the front row), let me remind you of your endocrine system and the main hormones that your amazing body produces.

The Endocrine System

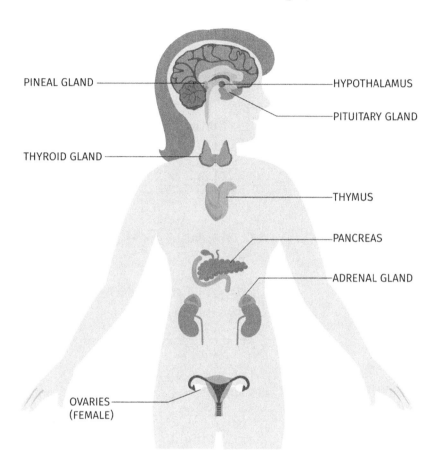

PINEAL GLAND

HYPOTHALAMUS

PITUITARY GLAND

THYROID GLAND

THYMUS

PANCREAS

ADRENAL GLAND

OVARIES
(FEMALE)

Hormones produced:

Pineal gland:	Melatonin – the hormone that helps you sleep
Pituitary gland:	TSH – thyroid stimulating hormone – stimulates thyroid hormones FSH – follicle stimulating hormone – prepares egg for release

	LH – luteinizing hormone – stimulates ovulation Growth hormone – stimulates growth, cell division and repair
Thyroid gland:	T4 (thyroxine) – primary thyroid hormone T3 (triiodothyronine) – active thyroid hormone
Pancreas:	Insulin and glucagon – regulate blood sugar levels
Adrenal glands:	Cortisol, adrenaline, DHEA – stress hormones
Ovaries:	Oestrogen, progesterone, testosterone – reproductive hormones

Melatonin – your SLEEP hormone

This is the hormone that is busy regulating your internal body clock and helping you get a good night's sleep. It's also a potent antioxidant and thought to protect against heart disease, cancer, diabetes and hormonal imbalances. It's made from the amino acid tryptophan (which you can get from most food protein sources), which converts to serotonin, then melatonin. So you need to be eating tryptophan in your diet (protein) and for the conversion to happen the brain needs to believe it's time for bed (i.e. total darkness!). That could be why it's also called the 'vampire hormone'!

Adrenaline, cortisol and DHEA – your STRESS hormones

Adrenaline
This is your major danger hormone, the one you feel coursing through you when someone jumps out at you, or when you narrowly avoid an oncoming car. It gets released from the adrenal glands in seconds once the brain recognizes that you're in potential danger. It's there to save you, but quickly disappears.

Cortisol
Cortisol takes a bit longer to get released (minutes rather than seconds). It has to go through a process called the HPA, the hypothalamic-pituitary-adrenal axis. And it's designed to prolong your 'fight or flight' state, in order to keep the body on alert, keep blood sugar high for energy, suppress any non-urgent functions and protect you from any further danger.

DHEA (Dehydroepiandrosterone)
DHEA is abundant when you're young but declines rapidly as you get older – it's often referred to as the 'youth hormone' for this reason. It helps to regulate insulin (reducing the risk of diabetes), improve mood and memory, and supports a healthy immune system. DHEA is often suppressed when you are stressed, as the adrenals prioritize the production of cortisol. However, DHEA can remain high in women with PCOS.

Insulin and glucagon – your BLOOD SUGAR regulators

Insulin
Insulin's life-saving job is to regulate your blood sugar. Too much sugar in your blood and you die, so it's vital for it to be controlled. Insulin is released from the pancreas when sugar enters the blood, either through eating it or through cortisol's actions when you are stressed. It takes the sugar out of the blood and carries it to your liver and to cells throughout the body. Your cells use it to

produce energy but any excess is taken to the liver and fat cells for storage. It's essentially a **fat-storing** hormone and can cause long-term health issues if it's out of balance.

Glucagon

Glucagon is the hormone that does the opposite to insulin. When blood sugar drops too low, the pancreas releases glucagon to signal to the liver to convert stored glucose (glycogen) back into glucose so that it can restore blood sugar levels to a safe level. When stored glucose is low, it tells fat cells to release fat to convert to sugar. So it's essentially your **fat-burning** hormone.

T4 and T3 – Thyroid hormones – your METABOLISM regulators

Your thyroid's life-saving job is to make every cell in your body work! Thyroid hormones are released from the thyroid gland and travel to every cell in the body. They control how much energy the cell produces, which can affect almost every process in the body from your heart beating to conceiving a baby. Thyroid hormones have their own pathway – the HPT (hypothalamus, pituitary, thyroid), and it depends on many factors being in place for it to work optimally.

Oestrogen, progesterone, testosterone – your SEX hormones

The oestrogens

Oestrogen is actually a group name for the three types: oestrone (E1), oestradiol (E2) and oestriol (E3). Oestrone is produced mainly after the menopause, oestradiol from puberty up to menopause and oestriol mainly during pregnancy. Oestradiol is the most potent oestrogen and is the one we produce mostly in our pre-menopausal years in our ovaries. It signals to the ovaries to ovulate, and builds up the uterine lining in preparation for an implanted fertilized egg. Oestrogens have many more functions in the body from maintaining healthy bones to keeping your skin supple and your brain sharp.

Progesterone

Progesterone's main function is to help the body prepare for and hold on to pregnancy. Produced in the ovaries during the second half of your cycle, it helps to prepare the uterus for an implanted egg. It prevents the uterine lining getting too thick, which can cause heavy periods. It also helps healthy cells to develop, reducing chances of uncontrolled cell division (which can lead to cancer). It is also produced in the adrenal glands and helps to calm you, balancing the stimulatory effect of oestrogen in the brain, helping to reduce anxiety and improve sleep quality. Progesterone also helps to support your thyroid hormones (boosting your metabolism), to lower insulin and boost your happy hormones serotonin and dopamine.

Testosterone

Testosterone is not just a male hormone. Women need it too for sex drive, heart health, energy, bone health, muscle mass and a sense of well-being and confidence. In women it is produced mainly in the adrenal glands, which if under any stress will prioritize the production of cortisol over sex hormones. Testosterone also declines rapidly with age (in both men and women), unless you have PCOS in which case it may still remain high. For the majority, by the time you hit 40, testosterone is half as much as it was in your 20s!

Your hormone journey – what happens as you age

I've decided that our bodies have some kind of 40-year warranty…

For the first 40 years we can live how we like (within reason!), eat and drink what we want and unless we have a particular genetic disposition we will usually be OK. After 40, however, the warranty has definitely run out! Unless we look after ourselves, we will be in and out of the garage with varying degrees of damage!

Your 20s

From puberty and into your 20s, oestrogen, progesterone and testosterone are in great shape, getting you ready to have a baby (whether you want one or not!). Your energy, sex drive, stress resilience and mental ability are high. You find it easy to lose weight and get fit. Your body is young and strong enough to cope with life's stressors. However, your lifestyle and environment can start to put a burden on your hormones at this age:

- toxins – alcohol, caffeine, drugs, smoking, environmental toxins, food chemicals – can all put a burden on the liver (which detoxifies excess oestrogen)
- poor diet – processed foods, trans-fats and low nutrients can affect how hormones function
- birth control pill – synthetic hormones alter your production of natural hormones and therefore can produce side effects such as mood swings, weight gain, insomnia, depression, headaches, fatigue and more
- environmental oestrogens – they are lurking in products like plastic and fragrance and can increase the risk of PMS, fibroids, endometriosis and breast or ovarian cancer
- excess stress – can affect digestion, immunity, weight, sexual function, fertility

But in your 20s generally your body is super resilient and can cope with a lot before showing any strain.

Your 30s

Your cycle should still be pretty regular, but your hormones are starting a gradual decline and may tip out of balance, especially if you've had children. If you have been through pregnancy your hormones increase, however after childbirth they can drop dramatically for a time causing mood swings and fatigue.

- Natural decline in progesterone can increase oestrogen dominance (PMS, poor sleep, fatigue, declining sex drive, PCOS, fibroids, endometriosis)
- Stress hormones are working harder – you might be juggling family, career, parents, partnerships, friends
- Poor diet – too many processed foods, refined carbohydrates, trans-fats, alcohol – can all contribute to weight gain, digestive issues, hormone imbalance
- More toxic accumulation – longer exposure to toxins, as well as your liver becoming less efficient means that toxins can accumulate (usually in your fat cells)
- Thyroid can weaken under the pressure of our stressful lives, or pregnancy – slowing our metabolism, reducing energy levels and making it harder to lose weight
- Digestive system may be feeling the impact of wear and tear, poor diet, toxins and stress

You still might not have any symptoms at this stage, but your resilience can start to weaken and you may notice subtle changes in your energy levels, weight and libido.

Your 40s

By your 40s, things can get really tricky – you are officially entering **perimenopause**, where your ovaries are coming to the end of their usefulness (ouch!).

- Progesterone levels are falling rapidly as you ovulate less regularly, so although oestrogen may be declining too, it's falling at a slower rate, so you are more likely to be oestrogen dominant – the list of symptoms is long, but includes PMS, irregular periods, mood swings, insomnia, anxiety, hot flushes, night sweats, low libido, low energy, vaginal dryness, urinary infections, joint pain, fibroids, brain fog and forgetfulness
- Your stress hormones may have been raging for some time, making you tired, overweight, anxious, unable to sleep and moody
- Your thyroid may be struggling to cope, making you feel exhausted, depressed, overweight, constipated, sluggish and cold. You might be losing your hair and your nails might be brittle
- You may have now built up quite a store of toxins putting a burden on your liver (so it's harder to detox your hormones properly, allowing them to recirculate)
- Diet choices tend to be ruled by low energy levels and blood sugar dips – coffee, carbs, sugary snacks – just to keep going
- Your digestive and immune functions can start to weaken (food intolerances, leaky gut, frequent infections, indigestion)
- Inflammation and oxidative stress are building (both increase risk of chronic disease)

Life might be a real struggle at this stage, or you may be sailing through with no problem (if you're one of the lucky ones!). If you are suffering, this is where some simple diet and lifestyle tweaks can make a big difference.

Your 50s

The average age for official menopause (when your periods have stopped completely for one whole year) is around 52. You've run out of eggs, which also means your hormones will never quite be the same again (this is fine if you are healthy!).

- All sex hormones (oestrogen, progesterone, testosterone) are generally at a much lower level – this can lead to wrinkles, dry skin, low libido, vaginal dryness, weight gain, poor bone and heart health, cognitive decline, hot flushes, night sweats and joint pain
- Stress – this decade can be stressful if you have a demanding job, marital issues, family, elderly parents or other psychological stresses (such as bereavement) – this can exacerbate menopausal symptoms
- Slow metabolism – a sluggish thyroid, less exercise and a natural decrease in your muscle tissue tend to slow the metabolism even more, increasing fatigue, brain fog and/or weight gain
- Long-term poor dietary and lifestyle habits may be taking their toll now, with higher risk of chronic conditions such as diabetes, heart disease, osteoporosis, dementia, arthritis and cancer

Many of the symptoms we put down to growing older – fatigue, joint pain, anxiety, insomnia, weight gain, low libido – can be due to hormonal decline. If you haven't started paying attention to your diet and lifestyle by now, it's definitely time! This is when putting up with continuing hormone imbalances can significantly increase your risk of more serious chronic conditions as you get older.

Let's face it, there's no doubt as you get older that your body is not going to be able to cope with the same things it did when you were younger. That piece of chocolate cake is going to have consequences that you didn't have to worry about when you were in your 20s.

But as long as you know how to look after yourself properly, you can still have the occasional treat and make those years beyond 40 and 50 the most happy and healthy possible.

Menopause and perimenopause
You don't officially reach menopause until one year after your last period. Perimenopause is the transition phase leading up to the menopause, which can start in your mid 30s.

What exactly is hormone balance?

The hormone symphony

Hormones work together in an incredibly complex system. They communicate with each other and are affected by one or more hormones being out of balance.

If for example you are particularly stressed over a period of time, this could slow down your thyroid function and also affect your sex hormone production. Equally, too much oestrogen can inhibit thyroid function and also weaken your adrenals.

Think about hormones like musicians in an orchestra. When they play together, the sound produced can be good or pretty awful. Individual musicians need to work together to make a great sound. If one or more are out of tune, too loud or quiet, then the whole sound suffers. What we want to hear is like a symphony; what we often hear is a cacophony!

What does hormone balance look like?

Symptoms of hormone imbalance can creep up on you very gradually – and it's easy to forget how you used to feel! So for me, being balanced means:

- having enough energy to be really productive at work, to enjoy exercise, and have enough left to go out for the evening occasionally!
- going shopping for clothes and knowing that they're going to fit
- being happy, calm and optimistic all through the month – and if you still have periods, not knowing when they're due other than what's in the calendar!
- glowing skin, healthy hair and nails
- getting deep restorative sleep every night
- having a clear, focused mind and memory

AND it means lower risk of more serious hormone-driven and other chronic health conditions down the line.

Does that sound impossible?

Well I thought so too… when I was going through my hormone issues I actually thought it was just a part of 'getting older' and I had to put up with it.

But it isn't as hard as you may think and this is what the book is all about…

SUMMARY

- Hormones are misunderstood and underestimated!
- Hormones control how we look, feel, think and behave
- It's important to know your key hormones and what they do

- Hormone imbalance can happen at any age beyond puberty
- Perimenopause is the transition between reproductive years and menopause (on average from 35 to 52)
- Hormones work together in a very delicate symphony
- Hormone balance is totally possible for you.

CHAPTER 2

TAKE THE QUIZ – FIND OUT IF YOU HAVE A HORMONE IMBALANCE

So firstly, you need to know if you even have a hormone imbalance, right?

You may feel you're too young, or your doctor may have told you there's nothing wrong (or offered you an antidepressant like mine did). But by looking at common symptoms, you may be surprised to find that it could be your hormones at fault.

In Chapter 1, I talked about the main symptoms of hormone imbalance that women experience in their 40s. If you want to know which ones you might have, take this short quiz and jump to the relevant chapters.

You can find this quiz in your accompanying workbook, which you can download and complete online at www. happyhormonesforlife.com/book.

The questionnaire is not designed to diagnose you. It is just a tool to give you an indication of whether you may have a hormonal imbalance and how you can help yourself using the Happy Hormone Code. I fully recommend you get personalized advice from a qualified medical or health practitioner if you have any serious conditions or want to get tested so you can implement a personalized programme (visit www.happyhormonesforlife. com/contact for more info).

Many of the symptoms in each part are the same and you may find that you have symptoms in more than one area. That's really common as hormones are so interwoven and one hormone out of whack will affect the others too. Usually there is one area that is the most dominant, and once you have addressed it, it often balances out the others. However, you may need to address all areas if your symptoms overlap.

The quiz

Rate the below symptoms from 0 to 3: 0 = does not occur, 1 = slight or occasional occurrence, 2 = moderate or common occurrence, 3 = severe and frequent occurrence.

Part 1 – Cortisol

1 Feeling wired/overwhelmed
1 Energy slumps during the day
1 Poor sleep
1 Anxious
2 Can't switch off
1 Mood swings, irritability
3 Low libido
0 Infertility
3 Fat around the middle (belly fat)
1 Salt or sugar cravings
0 Frequent colds/infections

Part 2 – Insulin

1 High waist:hip ratio (>0.8) (waist measurement divided by hip measurement)
1 Sleepy in the afternoon
1 Feeling 'hangry' (hungry/angry)
1 Dizzy or irritable before eating
2 Early hours insomnia (wake around 3–5)

PMS
ı Excessive thirst/or frequent urination
ı Sugar/carb cravings or carb-heavy diet

Part 3 – Thyroid

ı Fatigue (all day)
ı Weight gain
ı Depression
ı Anxiety
○ Dry or puffy skin/brittle nails
○ Hair loss
ı Low libido or infertility
2 Cold hands/feet
ı Brain fog, memory loss
ı PMS
ı Outer third of eyebrows missing
○ Constipation
○ High cholesterol
○ Family history of thyroid conditions

Part 4 – Low oestrogen

ı Hot flushes/night sweats
○ Dry itchy skin
ı Vaginal dryness
○ Deep wrinkles
ı Memory loss / brain fog
ı Low libido or painful sex
ı Tearfulness
ı Mood swings
2 Weight gain (belly, hips, thighs)

Part 5 – High oestrogen (or low progesterone)

3 Breast tenderness
o Heavy or painful periods
ı Water retention
' Mood swings
3 Acne
Σ Anxiety
o Fibroids, PCOS, endometriosis

Note your scores from each section in your notebook, or in the accompanying workbook. You can revisit this questionnaire when you have made some changes to see how your symptoms have improved.

If you have three or more symptoms in any one part then you are likely suffering a HORMONE IMBALANCE!

If you are dominant in Part 1 – jump to Chapter 3 for the low-down on **cortisol** OR straight to Chapter 7 for the Happy Hormone Code for what to do about it.

If you are dominant in Part 2 – jump to Chapter 3 for the low-down on **insulin** OR straight to Chapter 7 for the Happy Hormone Code for what to do about it.

If you are dominant in Part 3 – jump to Chapter 3 for the low-down on **thyroid** OR straight to Chapter 7 for the Happy Hormone Code for what to do about it.

If you are dominant in Part 4 or 5 – jump to Chapter 3 for the low-down on **oestrogen** OR straight to Chapter 7 for the Happy Hormone Code for what to do about it.

If you have symptoms in all 5 parts – please start the Happy Hormone Code immediately!

Medical Red Flags

While I'm speaking here about general symptoms of hormone imbalance, it is vital that you seek medical opinion if you have any of the following specific symptoms:

Pain

- any pain which is persistent, particularly if severe or in the head, abdomen or central chest
- pain in the eye or temples, with local tenderness, if you are elderly and/or rheumatic
- cystitis recurring more than three times in 12 months

Bleeding

- blood in sputum, vomit, urine or stools
- vomit containing 'coffee grounds'
- black, tarry stools
- non-menstrual vaginal bleeding (intermenstrual, postmenopausal, or at any time in pregnancy)
- vaginal bleeding with pain in pregnancy or after missing one period

Psychological

- deep depression with suicidal ideas
- hearing voices
- delusional beliefs
- uncharacteristic behaviour

Persistent

- vomiting and/or diarrhoea
- thirst
- increase in passing urine

- cough or hoarseness
- a sore that won't heal
- unexplained loss of weight (1lb per week or more)

Sudden

- breathlessness
- swelling of face, lips, tongue or throat
- blueness of the lips
- loss of consciousness
- loss of vision
- convulsions
- unexplained behavioural change

Difficulty

- swallowing
- breathing

Change

- in bowel habit
- in a skin lesion or mole (size, shape, colour, bleeding, itching, pain)

Others

- pallor
- unexplained swelling or lumps
- neck stiffness with fever
- unexplained fever, particularly if persistent or recurrent
- brown patches on the skin.

Mind the Gap

<u>Grab your notebook or workbook and complete the answers in the Mind the Gap section.</u>

If you've just taken the quiz and realized that you do have a hormone imbalance (or several!), please just take a moment to think about how it's affecting you and your life.

The reason I'm asking you to do this is that it really helps to know exactly where you are now, so you can work out where you want to be instead.

So take a moment to ask yourself these questions:

- Are you low in confidence?
- Is fatigue stopping you doing things?
- How are your moods affecting your relationships?
- How does stress make you feel?
- Is brain fog affecting your work?
- Are you having embarrassing hot flushes?
- How do other symptoms affect your life?
- What does all this stop you doing?

And now I'd like to ask you to take a moment to think about where you want to be. Without knowing your destination it's quite hard to know where you're going and when you are there!

So, take a moment to answer these questions:

- How do you want your body to look?
- How do you want to feel?
- How would that affect your life?
- What would that enable you to start doing?
- Who would that enable you to start being?

This last question was the one that really got me started. I didn't want to be the Grumpy Mum any more, I wanted to be Fun Mum…!

If there's a gap between where you are now, and where you want to be, all that you need is INFORMATION and a bit of SUPPORT.

Your big WHY

One of the keys to success in my programmes (and any programme that involves cultivating new habits) is motivation. This is the thing that goes out of the window very easily when things get tough. You've had a bad day at work, you have an argument with someone or you just haven't got the energy to keep going. That's when you need to call on your big WHY.

> **John Durant in his book *The Paleo Manifesto* says this:**
> *Leading a healthy lifestyle is a two-pronged problem; 1) knowing what's healthy, and 2) doing what's healthy. Science has focused on the first – figuring out what's healthy while neglecting the second – motivating people to make healthy decisions. The prescriptions of our diet culture, based on reductionist science, just aren't meaningful to most people. Vitamins never got anyone out of bed in the morning. There is something missing from our diets, and it's not a macronutrient or a vitamin. It's something deeper: meaning. Meaning is the secret ingredient that turns a diet into a lifestyle. So find ways to care about what you eat.*

Why do you want to sort out your hormones? This will be a bigger reason than you first think. You need a really big reason to make any changes in your life, especially diet and lifestyle! So many things and people are waiting for you to fail at this, so you need a damn good reason that will keep you going when things get tough. Life will get in the way (it's hard to eat well when you're really stressed, or unhappy or just exhausted) and people can be really unhelpful (they don't want you to show up their own inadequacies). So find your big reason and you will have the motivation to stick to your guns.

What is your WHY?

There are several layers to this answer. Let me explain with this example.

Answer 1 – 'I don't want to feel tired any more'

WHY?

Answer 2 – 'I want more energy to get more done during the day'

WHY?

Answer 3 – 'I want to start my own business'

WHY?

Answer 4 – 'I want to do something I really love and help others'

WHY?

Answer 5 – 'I want my family to be proud of me and my life to have been worth something'

Do you see how it takes a while to get down to the real reason you want to change? That's what you're looking for – that's your WHY and that will keep you going on the days where you want to give up.

When you've found your WHY, write it in your notebook or in the workbook. Then list 50 things you will be able to get out of improving your hormone health. Get that list out every time you have a slip-up or a bad day, and start again.

My own WHY for hormone health is unashamedly selfish, actually. I love travelling and there are so many places I want to see. I want to visit them all and to do that I need boundless energy and enthusiasm. I want to spend my retirement with a suitcase in my hand! This motivates me to look after my body and mind. I won't be going anywhere if I'm exhausted and moody (I won't have a husband to go with either!).

If you don't have a WHY, then your chances of successfully improving your health are low I'm afraid. Go back over the questions until you can't answer 'why' any more.

Your main goals

Once you've got your big WHY, you can create some juicy goals to go with it. List them in your notebook or workbook.

SUMMARY

Identify which of your hormones may be out of balance:
- cortisol
- insulin
- thyroid
- low or high oestrogen
- a mix of all of these

Be clear on the main issues you want to resolve and identify and write down your big juicy goals!

CHAPTER 3

MEET YOUR FEISTY 4

Out of the 100 or so hormones that are swimming around your body, there are four major ones that pretty much dictate how you look, feel, think and perform. I call them the 'Feisty 4' as they really can be tricky to control, especially after the age of 40. Unless you are looking after them, they can sabotage your weight-loss efforts, keep your metabolism on hold, crash your energy levels and cause hormone mayhem!

Let me introduce you…

THE FEISTY 4

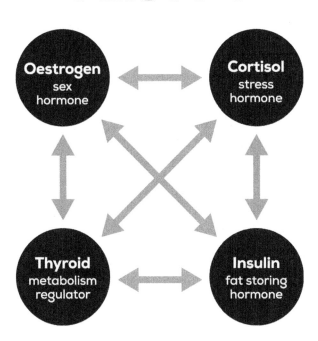

1 – Cortisol – your STRESS hormone

The hormone behind many stress-related issues is cortisol. Its job is to keep you alive, so it's pretty damn important! Cortisol is released from the adrenal glands to wake you up in the morning, keep you alert during the day and help you manage any dangers or threats that come your way.

In caveman times, stress hormones saved your life from a lion attack or a famine. Your 'fight or flight' response would kick in – the brain would send a message to the adrenals to release adrenaline (the big initial rush), and cortisol (to keep you on high alert).

These hormones:

- raise blood sugar levels (so that you can run away fast)
- stimulate insulin release (to get the sugar into your muscle cells)
- raise blood pressure so oxygen can get to the muscles quicker (so you can run away fast)
- mobilize stored fat into the abdomen area to protect vital organs in case of attack (and provide quick energy so you can run away fast)
- break down muscle, skin and bone to make more sugar (so that you can run away fast)
- suppress immunity (fighting off an infection is not a priority when you need to run)
- suppress digestion (no need to digest food when your life is in danger)
- suppress reproductive function (hence lack of libido – who needs sex drive when you are under attack?)

You get the picture. A really important life-saving mechanism when you're being chased by a lion. Not quite so useful when you're sitting in a traffic jam, or feeling overwhelmed!

Of course, you still need your 'fight or flight' response for emergencies, but these days, it's modern-day stresses like demanding bosses, deadlines, relationship issues, traffic jams, kids, money worries and more, that switch it on.

Unfortunately, Mother Nature only gave you ONE stress response. That's the 'fight or flight' one that evolved to keep you alive. I guess she couldn't imagine a time when we would have 24/7 technology, long working hours and the other modern-day stresses that we all face.

Your brain is an amazing thing. But it can't distinguish between a real danger (lion) and a perceived danger (traffic jam). Either way, your body reacts as if you're being attacked and you might die.

Why your evolutionary stress response can be problematic:

It's designed to be **temporary** – once you escaped or killed the lion, you could rest in your cave and recover. You can't escape from modern-day stresses – there is no rest and recover time – it's unrelenting.

All that **sugar** mobilized for energy to fight or run from your source of stress isn't being used up (unless you go kick-boxing after work every day) – so it gets stored as FAT – usually around the middle where it can be easily accessed.

Cortisol has **priority** over everything. When you are in danger, all your reserves are diverted to survival mechanisms. That means no energy for:

- digestive processes – digesting and absorbing vital nutrients
- fat burning – your metabolism is stalled to conserve energy and fat stores

- immunity – fighting infection and toxins
- sex hormones – reproduction, monthly cycle, sex drive, bone health

Your body has evolved and adapted in many ways since caveman times, but your adrenal stress response is exactly the same.

Sources of stress

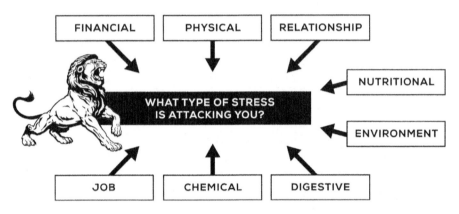

You may think of stress as the feeling of overwhelm when you've got a lot on your plate. But it's not just the obvious things that put a stress on your body. There are many potential stressors that you may not even be aware of. Here are just a few:

- physical – trauma, illness, accident, surgery, ageing, allergies, inflammation, starvation
- emotional – grief, anger, guilt, bereavement, divorce, relationships, feeling insecure, unloved, fearful, anxious, lonely, overwhelmed, depressed
- dietary – alcohol, caffeine, sugar, trans-fats, refined carbs, food chemicals, nutrient deficiencies
- medications – anti-inflammatories, antacids, contraceptive pill, statins, etc.

- environmental – pollution, chemicals, toxins, extremes of temperature, noise
- lifestyle – smoking, drugs, prolonged sitting, over-exercise, poor sleep, shift work

Good stress

Don't get me wrong, a bit of stress in your life is a good thing. You need good stress: it keeps you alert and excited, it helps the body adapt, enhances your immune function, repairs your tissues and, more importantly, wakes you up in the morning! An example of good stress is exercise. You break down muscle when you work out, and this puts the body under stress. But the body repairs the damaged muscle with bigger and stronger tissue so that you can be better prepared the next time it happens. That's a very clever evolutionary process, don't you think? But it only works if you rest in between workouts. This gives the body time to heal and repair and build stronger muscle.

Adrenaline and cortisol make you feel alert and excited. But the feeling doesn't last long – these hormones will deplete you if you don't give yourself a chance to rest and repair afterwards. So that roller coaster ride will make you feel amazing, but not if you stay on it over and over. You need to recover before the next ride.

Bad stress

When you have managed to escape from or kill the lion, your stress is resolved and your hormones go back to normal. This is the normal physiological response that our bodies have cleverly developed for our own survival and it works brilliantly. But modern-day stress is not so easy. You can't run away from your boss or kill someone who's annoying you! So the stress often remains unresolved.

Whether you are trying to juggle family, career, exercise, relationships and social life, or whether you are battling with emotional issues, this unrelenting stress can cause your cortisol levels to remain high all the time. Cortisol gets to be the alpha male and run riot. All the other hormones then struggle to make themselves heard and you start to get symptoms of hormone imbalance (the cacophony).

Are you more stressed than you used to be?

There are a few reasons life can seem more stressful as you age.

1. Life actually IS more stressful! You may have:
    *   more senior roles at work or running your own business
    *   kids – likely to be teenagers
    *   relationship issues
    *   ageing parents – health issues or needing care
    *   bereavement of someone close
    *   money or debt worries
    *   loneliness
    *   health issues
    *   feelings of unfulfilment (midlife crisis)

2. Your hormonal efficiency and stress resilience declines so you can't deal with stress like you used to.

3. Your hormones are fluctuating all over the place during perimenopause, causing additional stress on the body.

Common symptoms

Wired/overwhelmed – Stress is often mistaken for being 'busy'. It's not actually about how busy you are, but about how you respond to it. When you feel overwhelmed, racing from one task to another, and find it hard to calm down or switch off – you are in a state of high alert. If you can't switch off the source of the stress, cortisol levels stay high and you can feel frazzled.

Cranky – Cortisol can interfere with your brain biochemistry, making you quick to feel angry, irritable and impatient. If you are snapping at everyone and want to kill the person in front of you because they are walking too slowly, this is a sign!

Mood swings – If you are lacking any motivation to get out of bed, you can't find any joy in life or you find yourself in tears for no apparent reason, it's a sign that cortisol could be messing with your neurotransmitters. Many studies have linked stress with depression and mood swings.

Belly fat – Will that spare tyre around your middle just not go, no matter what diet you try or how much exercise you do? If you have a hormone imbalance, you won't sustain weight loss no matter how hard you try. Not only do we have four times more cortisol receptors in our abdominal fat than any other part of the body, but cortisol also stimulates appetite – sugar and carbs are vital when you need energy to run from that lion. But when food is readily available and there is no lion to run from, the sugar you have eaten doesn't get used as energy and is stored away as fat. Your blood sugar surge has increased insulin levels (your fat-storing hormone), leading to a blood sugar crash, and another uncontrollable craving for a biscuit, pastry or bar of chocolate. And the exhausting cycle goes on…

Energy slumps – Whether your cortisol levels are high or low, it will take a toll on your energy levels. If they are high and you are under chronic stress, it will be hard for your blood sugar to stay in balance and the dips will make you feel tired. This often happens in the afternoon – cravings for sugar, coffee and carbs are especially common at this time. That afternoon cake or chocolate run? Now it makes sense. Your body is low on sugar and is sending you a powerful message: 'feed me sugar or I will send you off to sleep!' If you are low in cortisol, you might find it hard to even get out of bed in the morning and just feel exhausted all day.

Poor sleep – If you're stressed during the day, it can really disrupt your sleep patterns. If you are up late checking emails, social media or working late into the night, you can have trouble switching off when you need to get to sleep. Or often you wake up at 3am because your blood sugar is low and it stimulates a cortisol release. So you wake up unrefreshed, you reach for the coffee or sugary cereal to wake you up – and the whole blood sugar cycle starts again!

Anxious – Cortisol feeds your anxieties. If you're in a state of alert, expecting imminent death/danger, your mind will be racing. Your heightened senses may manifest as worry, fear, nervousness or panic. Of course, good stress can provide a source of extreme excitement (think skydiving). But good stress is always followed by rest and repair (you don't skydive continuously!).

Brain fog/memory loss – Brain fog or memory lapses affect many people when they're stressed. Think interview situations or exams – how easy is it to forget something important just because you're under pressure? Cortisol is messing with your neurotransmitters, and if you are perimenopausal this can get a whole lot worse.

Digestive issues – You know that sick feeling in your gut when you are stressed or anxious? We have more nerve cells in our gut than in our brain – after all, this is where our 'gut instinct' comes from. Emotions and stress are felt in this area and this can seriously impair your digestion. Cortisol doesn't care about digesting food when you're facing a lion, so it shuts much of the system down. That's why you can have 'butterflies', nausea or diarrhoea just before that big presentation. When the stress continues however, you're stuck with dodgy digestion long term.

Frequent colds/infections – Why do you always pick up a cold or infection the minute you relax or go on holiday? High cortisol rapidly depletes your vitamin C stores, along with your B vitamins and essential minerals. It also reduces the production of immune cells, leaving you more vulnerable to infection. And if your vitamin D is low too, you'll be very lucky to avoid the lurgy!

Low sex drive and/or infertility – Stress and reproduction? They really don't go together! Cortisol dampens down your sex hormones, so no wonder you reach for the chocolate bar instead of your partner. Cortisol and the sex hormones are all made from the same precursor hormone, pregnenolone. So guess what happens when you are stressed? Pregnenolone gets the message to make more cortisol instead of sex hormones (as we know that our stress response takes priority over our reproductive function when we need to run away). Cortisol also increases another hormone, prolactin, which can stop you ovulating. So your sex hormones take a back seat, your testosterone and libido disappear, and forget about getting pregnant. Sensibly the body is trying to protect you. It doesn't want you bringing a baby into a 'dangerous' world.

PMS – Cortisol competes with progesterone, so the more stressed you are, the less progesterone you are likely to make. As progesterone balances out oestrogen, this can lead to oestrogen dominance and PMS symptoms such as mood swings, cramps, heavy periods, bloating and breast tenderness.

Hot flushes – Stress and cortisol can be a common trigger for hot flushes and night sweats during the peri- and post-menopausal years.

Adrenal fatigue or burn out – Constantly high cortisol levels are sustainable for varying degrees of time. Some people are stress bunnies for years and years, and may be able to function fine on it. Others can keep going for some time until they get adrenal dysfunction or cortisol resistance. This is where the adrenal organs that are pumping out all this cortisol and adrenaline get overwhelmed and can't keep up with demand, or where cell receptors for cortisol are worn out and stop functioning, making that cell 'resistant' to the cortisol trying to get in.

Either way, you are going to slow down rapidly. Your cortisol levels may be low all day long, potentially causing serious fatigue, muscle aches, frequent infections, digestive problems and low mood. This is often called 'burn out' or 'adrenal fatigue'. It is not a condition generally recognized by conventional medicine, as the only treatments available are for the extreme high and low of adrenal function (very high cortisol is Cushing's syndrome, extreme low is Addison's disease). Both these conditions are very serious and require immediate treatment. Test results that fall anywhere in between these extremes are classed as 'normal' or 'subclinical' manifestations and won't be treated.

High or low 'subclinical' cortisol levels, however, are not good states to be in. They both have consequences for hormone balance and can have debilitating symptoms that seriously impact on quality of life. You may be left wondering what on earth is wrong with you, or you may feel that nobody is taking you seriously. Unfortunately if the adrenals are not looked after, for some it can increase the risk of serious illness such as Chronic Fatigue Syndrome (or ME), depression, fibromyalgia, IBS, autoimmune conditions and some cancers.

To have any impact on your overall hormone balance, and to avoid potential adrenal fatigue, it's really important to get your cortisol under control.

Jump to Part 3 for more information.

Alice's story

A stress bunny

Alice is a 47-year-old city worker. She came to see us as she was stressed out, exhausted, could not shift her belly fat and was fed up that her wardrobe was dwindling – she couldn't fit into her slick city suits any more. So we needed to identify all her stressors and start balancing her cortisol and insulin. She started including 'hormone-friendly foods' in her diet (see p. 160). Within seven days, she had lost 3lbs and had more energy. Her brain fog had lifted and she was sleeping better. This is what she had to say:

'I just wanted to lose the belly fat that I couldn't shift with my usual low-calorie diet. By managing my stress and identifying any hidden stressors (in my case, it was sugar!), I was able to address the root cause of my weight loss resistance so that my body could release it. After 30 days I lost 10lbs of belly fat, and felt amazing! By understanding how my hormones work and how to get them working well, I now have full control over them, and my weight.'

SUMMARY

- Cortisol has priority over everything
- You only have one 'fight or flight' stress response
- It has to be switched off in order to work in your favour (see Chapter 8)
- Too much stress can make you tired, grumpy, fat, depressed, craving sugar and foggy (and crush your sex drive)
- Sustained high cortisol levels can lead to adrenal fatigue and/or chronic disease

---

Quick tips

1. **Put yourself first** – as women we don't do this enough. We give to everyone around us and wonder why we suffer!
2. **Prioritize rest and relaxation** – that means making sure nothing comes in the way of your relaxation time (and sleep). Have gadget-free days or limit the time you check your phone/email.
3. **Find something you love** – yoga, massage, meditation, long bath, whatever floats your boat – just do it!
4. **Breathe** – just the act of deep breathing from your belly switches off your cortisol response. How amazingly easy is that? You can do that in bed!
5. **Stop feeling guilty** – so many women feel guilty when relaxing. WHY? If you don't relax, everyone around you is going to suffer! Call it giving back…
6. **Nourish your adrenals** – make sure you are supplementing those nutrients that stress is depleting (vitamin C, B vitamins, magnesium, zinc) with a good quality multivitamin complex.

7. **Adaptogenic herbs** – these can help to balance cortisol levels – including rhodiola, ashwagandha, liquorice and American ginseng (always check with a qualified herbalist before using herbs).
8. **Balance your blood sugar** – avoid refined carbs and sugar, and eat low GL foods including organic fruit and vegetables, nuts, seeds, organic meat, fish and full-fat dairy products.
9. **Remove food stressors** – processed foods, sugar, vegetable oils, and suspected intolerances (e.g. gluten, dairy).
10. **Avoid caffeine and alcohol** – both of these can increase the burden on your adrenals.
11. **Don't do strenuous exercise if you are low on energy** – over-exercising can deplete your reserves – try gentle walking or yoga instead.

2 – Insulin – your fat-storing hormone

Will that spare tyre around your middle just not go, no matter what diet you try or how much exercise you do?

Insulin is one of the hormones responsible. It's your FAT-STORING HORMONE! You absolutely need insulin – it has a life-saving job of regulating your blood sugar levels, which need to be kept in a very narrow range, or it can be dangerous. But your diet and lifestyle can contribute to overly high levels of insulin, which can be problematic.

Insulin is released from your pancreas when you eat food containing sugar (not just sweet stuff, carbohydrates are just more complex sugars). Once the sugar is absorbed into your blood, insulin mops up the excess and takes it to the cells of your liver, muscles and fat to help move the glucose inside to use as energy. The liver and muscles take what they need and the rest is stored in your fat cells for future use.

Putting it really simply, the more insulin you produce, the more fat you tend to store. The more carbs and sugar you eat, the more insulin you produce. That's why high carb/sugar diets are generally the most fattening.

A spoonful of sugar

Dr Michael Eades in his blog 'A spoonful of sugar' explains that a normal amount of sugar in your blood (after fasting) is just less than a teaspoon (approx 4g). To be diagnosed as diabetic your fasting blood sugar only needs to have gone up to 6.25g – this is a teaspoon and a quarter – just a quarter of a teaspoon more than a 'normal' reading.

A portion of McDonald's fries contains 47g of carbs (= 47g of sugar), 10 teaspoons going into your blood. Getting all this sugar out of your blood is a huge task for your body already, but imagine adding in a giant Coke, a Big Mac and maybe an apple pie for dessert?! No wonder we have a diabetes epidemic.

Fat storing in caveman times was really important to protect against famine. This stored fat would protect you in leaner times against starvation. And there wasn't access to much sugar (the odd berry from a tree or some honey) so they didn't have the blood sugar swings that are daily occurrences in modern times. Unfortunately your body hasn't yet evolved to cope with food available 24/7!

The blood sugar roller coaster

When you eat too many carbs or you are majorly stressed, the resulting blood sugar surge stimulates large amounts of insulin, which in its super efficient job of removing the sugar can lead to a blood sugar crash a little while later (hypoglycaemia), and another uncontrollable craving for a biscuit, pastry or bar of chocolate. And here we go again…!

On a graph this looks like one of those crazy scary roller coasters and what you want to aim for is a nice gentle ride; more of a wavy line instead.

These are some of the things that can cause the blood sugar roller coaster:

- refined carbs – bread, pasta, white rice, rice cakes, biscuits, cereal, cakes, pastries

- sugar – fruit juice, honey, cordial, fizzy drinks, sugar of all kind (including agave nectar and honey)
- fruit – high sugar fruits include tropical fruit, bananas, pears etc.
- dried fruit – just like candy!
- skipping meals – can cause hypoglycaemia (low blood sugar)
- alcohol – a quick sugar release that stimulates cortisol and insulin
- artificial sweeteners – shown to stimulate insulin despite no actual 'sugar'
- caffeine (particularly on an empty stomach)
- stress – cortisol pumps sugar into your blood!

The Blood Sugar Rollercoaster

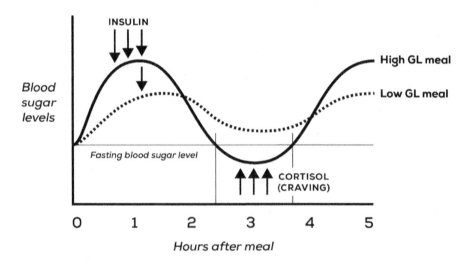

The stress connection

Low blood sugar sends a stress signal to the brain, resulting in cortisol being released to get sugar back into your blood. So even if you're on the best low-sugar/carb diet in the world, but you're stressed out, you'll still be on the blood sugar roller coaster, which itself is exhausting for your body, releasing more cortisol which puts more sugar into the blood to continue the vicious cycle...

But it's not just fat storing that we need to worry about...

Too much insulin can contribute to chronic diseases including:

- obesity
- diabetes
- inflammation
- osteoporosis
- dementia/Alzheimer's
- hormone imbalance
- thyroid disease
- PCOS and endometriosis
- digestive issues
- cancer
- heart disease

And on top of all this, it makes you AGE FASTER! All that sugar in the blood causes something called glycation – it sticks to proteins in your body and causes damage and ageing.

Common symptoms

High waist:hip ratio – the ratio of your waist circumference to your hip circumference (calculated by dividing the waist circumference by the hip circumference) should be less than 0.8 for women. Higher than this and it's an indication that your blood sugar may be out of balance and you're at an increased risk of insulin resistance and diabetes.

Sugar/carb cravings – if your blood sugar is unstable, you will have frequent highs and lows, and during those lows you are likely to have sugar or carb cravings to get your levels back to normal. The more carbs you eat, the more unstable your blood sugar, and round we go…

Early hours insomnia – the more carb heavy your diet (or stressed your day is), the more chance you could have blood sugar dips during the night, which can release cortisol and wake you up – usually around the 3am mark. That glass of wine at night to relax you? Or that late night chocolate snack? They might help to get you off to sleep but they can cause a blood sugar dip and wake you up in the early hours.

Afternoon slump – the 3–5pm afternoon slump is when you really want that nap! That's a blood sugar dip making you really tired. Usually from a bread- or carb-based lunch.

PMS – excess insulin can increase your oestrogen levels, leaving you susceptible to oestrogen dominant symptoms such as irritability, mood swings, bloating, cravings, breast tenderness and heavy periods.

Headaches, irritability, shakiness, poor concentration (relieved by eating) – if your blood sugar is low, your brain might not be functioning very well until you eat again.

Excessive thirst and/or frequent urination – when you have too much sugar in your blood, your kidneys need to work hard to remove it, resulting in frequent urination and feeling more thirsty than normal.

Family history of diabetes – you may have an inherited genetic susceptibility to poor blood sugar control, however this is not a life sentence! Your lifestyle has a huge impact on whether those inherited genes of yours get fully expressed.

To have any impact on your overall hormone balance, and to avoid future potential health conditions, it's really important to get your blood sugar and insulin under control.

Jump to Part 3 to find out more.

Amanda's story

A sugar addict

Amanda is a 45-year-old mum of three who came to see us to lose weight. She was a self-confessed sugar addict, and had cravings pretty much all day long. Sugar was ruling her life, and as a result her waistline. She was two stone overweight and gaining. Her energy was very low and she felt too sluggish to exercise. She had brain fog and mood swings and was desperate to regain control.

We suggested she started with some healthy smoothies, which filled her up til lunchtime and stopped her usual mid-morning craving for a cookie. Eating more fat and protein at lunchtime and dinner helped her balance her blood sugar and increase her metabolism. Here's what she said:

'I had tried every diet going and nothing worked. I couldn't seem to keep the willpower going to resist my chocolate and biscuit cravings. When I started following these principles, I was amazed at how quickly my cravings disappeared. The smoothies were so filling, I didn't have room for anything til lunchtime! And then all I craved were healthy foods that my body needed. I have lost 14lbs. I am still sugar-free and the fat is still dropping off me!'

SUMMARY

- Insulin is your 'fat-storing' hormone
- Stress and insulin are closely linked (they are bad for each other!)
- Eating too many carbs/sugar will put you on the blood sugar roller coaster (and once you're on, it's very hard to get off)
- Keeping your blood sugar stable (and insulin under control) is vital for hormone balance and weight control
- Too long on the blood sugar roller coaster and your risk of more serious conditions goes up

---

Quick tips

1. **Get off the roller coaster!** – Avoid processed sugary foods and choose slower release carbs like non-starchy vegetables, oats, brown rice, quinoa, beans, pulses, legumes.

2. **Eat protein with each meal (especially breakfast!).**

3. **Eat fat to lose fat** – fat blunts the insulin response from a meal, reducing the impact of the carbs.

4. **Watch the alcohol** – not only for its sugar content, but also for the bad choices it tends to encourage!

5. **Don't skip meals** – but don't over-snack either! Stick to three 'low GL' meals a day.

6. **Move more** – exercise helps insulin do its job effectively so we don't need as much.

7. **Add a teaspoon of cinnamon daily** – cinnamon has been shown to help to regulate blood sugar levels.

8. **Slow down and chill out** – too much cortisol will keep that tyre around your middle, and put you at higher risk of fatigue, heart disease, diabetes and cancer.

9. **Get enough sleep** – lack of sleep has been shown to increase appetite hormones. And when we're tired and stressed out, our healthy food choices go out the window.

10. **Supplements can be helpful** – magnesium, chromium, alpha lipoic acid, vitamin D, zinc, berberine and adaptogenic herbs have all shown potential benefits for blood sugar control. (Do check with your doctor or health practitioner before taking any new supplements.)

3 – Thyroid – your METABOLISM regulator

If you have a normally functioning thyroid, you may be a bit sceptical when you hear a woman with some extra weight blaming it on her thyroid. But thyroid conditions are absolutely real and becoming much more common, especially in women over 35. And if you have low levels of thyroid hormone it is extremely difficult to lose any weight – believe me I've been there!

You see, your thyroid hormones are vital for every cell in your body to function properly (every single cell has a thyroid receptor). Thyroid hormones are a bit like a thermostat for our cells. They either turn you up (increase your metabolism, energy, temperature, alertness) or they turn you down (slow down your metabolism, conserve energy, decrease temperature, shut down non-essential functions), depending on how much hormone you have available. If your thyroid hormone isn't functioning properly, it can affect almost everything, resulting in symptoms pretty much anywhere in the body.

Hypothyroidism (too little thyroid) is a lot more common than hyperthyroidism (too much thyroid), and mainly affects women over 35, due to genetic inheritance, the demands of pregnancy and the hormone imbalances we go through during the perimenopausal years.

The thyroid gland is a small butterfly-shaped organ in the base of your neck. Just like the adrenal hormone cascade, there is also one for the thyroid hormones. It's called the HPT – the hypothalamic-pituitary-thyroid axis:

Hypothalamic-Pituitary-Thyroid Axis

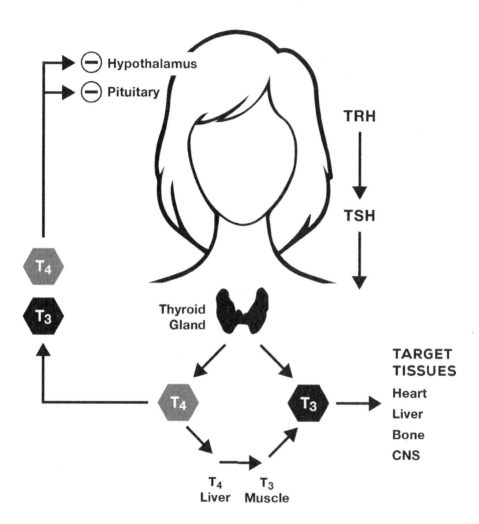

1. **TSH (thyroid stimulating hormone)** – is produced by the pituitary gland. Its job is to stimulate the thyroid to produce thyroxine (T4) and triiodothyronine (T3). When the levels of T4 and T3 in the body drop too low, the hypothalamus in the brain gets the message that we need more and signals to the pituitary gland to produce thyroid hormones. So TSH is the first marker to look at when assessing thyroid function

(high levels mean the body is trying to respond to low levels of thyroid in the body = potential hypothyroidism).

2. **T4 (thyroxine)** – is mainly a pro-hormone, i.e. it converts into either T3 or Reverse T3 (RT3).

3. **T3 (triiodothyronine)** – is the active thyroid hormone. Free T3 is typically elevated in hyperthyroidism and lowered in hypothyroidism.

4. **RT3 (Reverse T3)** is made by the body to tone down energy. If T3 is the accelerator, then RT3 is the handbrake. It stops the T3 hormone from signalling the cell to make energy. It allows the body to turn down the energy when it needs to. Elevated RT3 can result in hypothyroid symptoms.

So if for any reason you are not converting your T4 to T3 very well, or your RT3 is too high, your thyroid function will suffer, DESPITE your TSH readings. Which is why you may still have symptoms of low thyroid even if your TSH is normal.

These are some of the many functions of the thyroid hormones:

- regulate metabolism (how and what you burn for energy), therefore your weight
- stimulate fat burning and reduce cholesterol
- regulate temperature – stimulating energy (heat) production, keeping the body warm
- support brain function (memory, alertness, mood)
- support digestive system, keeping bowels moving and liver detoxing
- support reproductive health – fertility, libido and menstrual health
- support immune system to fight infection
- boost blood circulation, supplying oxygen and nutrients to cells

- keep skin soft and supple
- keep hair and nails strong and thick
- keep arteries clear, cholesterol down and regulates blood pressure
- keep muscles and joints lubricated and supple, bones strong
- prevent fluid retention (puffy face/eyes) and bloating
- prevent headaches

As you can see if you don't have enough thyroid hormones, it can affect almost any part of your body. On top of that if the thyroid is out of whack, you can bet your other hormones will be too. You can't be truly healthy if it goes untreated.

The production and function of your thyroid hormones depends on a range of nutrients as well as a healthy gut, liver, immune and hormonal system!

This book focuses on symptoms relating to LOW thyroid (hypothyroidism) as this is the most common imbalance, but you should also look out for HIGH thyroid (hyperthyroidism) – symptoms can include palpitations, bulging eyes, high blood pressure, sweating, diarrhoea, anxiety, weight loss. In either case, you need to get informed so you can discuss it fully with your doctor. Be aware however that many symptoms of hormone imbalance are similar, so you need to ask for all hormones to be tested.

Causes of hypothyroidism

Hashimoto's disease
The most common cause of hypothyroidism (especially in women over 40) is an autoimmune condition called Hashimoto's disease. This is where your immune system produces antibodies to your own thyroid gland, preventing it from functioning

properly. Presence of certain antibodies will confirm this; however testing is not 100% reliable.

Nutrient deficiency (including low calorie diets)

Production of T4 and T3 depends on many nutrients. If your diet is lacking in any of the following, you may not be able to produce enough hormones. Low thyroid also causes poor absorption of nutrients as it slows down your digestive system.

- Iodine – an integral part of the T4 and T3 molecule. Deficiency often manifests as a goitre – an enlargement of the thyroid gland. Iodine deficiency is much more prevalent than it used to be. Unless you are eating seafood and sea vegetables (or micro algae) fairly regularly you are probably not getting enough iodine. However, supplementation is controversial as too much iodine can also harm your thyroid! Check with your health practitioner and get your iodine levels tested before supplementing.
- Tyrosine – is the T part of the thyroid hormone molecule. This is an amino acid (breakdown of protein) so you need to be eating adequate protein.
- Minerals needed for conversion of T4 to T3:
  - selenium
  - copper
  - zinc.
- Iron is needed for efficient uptake of iodine.
- Vitamin A is needed for T3 to do its job in the cell.
- Vitamin C is important for regulating thyroid function.
- Vitamin D helps to regulate the immune system and reduce antibodies.

Stress and insulin

Cortisol can be either helpful or harmful to the thyroid. Too much or too little cortisol can interfere with the T4 to T3 conversion.

Cortisol can increase insulin, which has also been linked to low thyroid, so the circle is indeed vicious!

Low progesterone/high oestrogen

High levels of oestrogen can increase thyroid-binding proteins that can decrease the levels of free thyroid hormone. Progesterone is needed for the conversion of T4 to T3.

Food intolerances

One of the causes of Hashimoto's disease can be food intolerances. The most common foods to cause an autoimmune reaction are gluten and dairy. Gluten sensitivity or full-blown coeliac disease has been linked to Hashimoto's. If you are sensitive to gluten or dairy, you can develop a 'leaky gut' or intestinal permeability where the lining of the gut lets in undigested food particles, bacteria or toxins that travel in your blood causing damage to organs and tissues. The thyroid gland is particularly vulnerable to attack, as the molecular composition of thyroid tissue is almost identical to that of gluten – which is why your immune system attacks your thyroid as well as the gluten – a case of mistaken identity.

Toxins

A wide range of environmental agents has been found to interfere with thyroid hormone (and hormones in general – see Chapter 4). Plastics, pollutants, pesticides, heavy metals and many other chemicals can block the uptake of iodine, and increase the risk of autoimmune attack.

Exposure to chlorine (mainly through showering and tap water), fluoride (toothpaste) and bromine (in some baked goods) can also interfere with the thyroid receptors on the cells.

Radiation

Exposure to radiation from X-rays and radiation therapy can inhibit iodine uptake to make thyroid hormones.

Goitrogenic foods

These are foods that can antagonize the thyroid gland. These include soy, millet, peanuts and raw cruciferous vegetables (broccoli, cauliflower, Brussels sprouts, cabbage, kale, rocket, chard, watercress etc) – although indications are that you need to be eating large quantities of these foods in their raw form for them to have a disrupting effect. Cooking them neutralizes any negative effects.

Pregnancy

Some women develop hypothyroidism during or after pregnancy. The demand for thyroid hormones from the growing baby increases throughout pregnancy. Thyroid antibodies can also be produced and impair thyroid function.

Family history

Thyroid problems do have strong genetic factors.

Common symptoms

Weight gain – if you're overweight and can't lose it no matter what you eat, your thyroid may be the culprit. Low thyroid means slower metabolism – less fat burning and more fat storage. It will be nearly impossible to lose weight when you have an underactive thyroid, and your energy levels make it difficult to exercise.

Fatigue – constant exhaustion can be a sign that your thyroid is slowing down your system to conserve energy. This can result in feeling tired even if you have had a good night's sleep. If your adrenals are stressed then you may not be getting the best quality sleep anyway, adding to the exhaustion.

Mood swings, anxiety or depression – low thyroid has long been associated with depression and mood swings. Thyroid hormones affect serotonin levels and regulate oxygen uptake by brain cells.

Brain fog/memory loss – if your brain cells aren't able to produce enough energy, they will slow right down and fog up your thinking. Brain cells have more T3 receptors than any other parts of the body!

Constipation – low thyroid can cause your digestion to slow down, which can result in bloating and constipation. Slow circulation and metabolism means that cells are slow to get rid of their waste products, leaving you with a puffy face and/or eyes.

Cold – you're the only one that is wearing a jumper and socks in bed? A slower metabolism will slow down your circulation and make you less tolerant to cold, especially in your hands and feet.

Hair loss, dry skin, flaky nails – thinning hair, dry cracked skin and poor nails are often due to slow circulation and metabolism. If you are missing the outer third of your eyebrows, this is another sign of low thyroid (not diagnostic, just an indicator).

Low sex drive and infertility – thyroid hormones regulate your sex hormone production. If you don't have enough thyroid your sex drive can plummet and fertility can be affected. Thyroid also helps convert cholesterol into progesterone, essential for a healthy pregnancy.

PMS – thyroid hormones regulate sex hormone production and the menstrual cycle. Low thyroid can result in irregular, heavy or painful periods, bloating, headaches, mood swings and fatigue.

Some of these symptoms are similar to those resulting from stress and oestrogen imbalances. That's because your adrenal, thyroid and sex hormone function are closely interconnected. An imbalance in one is likely to affect the other. It's important to check all sets of symptoms, see your doctor or a health practitioner and get yourself tested. Your adrenal health needs to be prioritized, as nothing else will improve unless this is resolved.

Jump to Chapter 10 for information on what tests are available both with your GP and privately. Unfortunately the symptoms of low thyroid (weight gain, depression, fatigue) are often brushed aside as an age thing. Don't accept that you are just 'getting old'. If you've got this far in the book already, then you know that this is not an excuse.

If you want to do an easy test at home that can give you an indication of whether your thyroid is sluggish, there is one called the Barnes Basal Test. This involves taking your temperature on waking for six days (see the Resources section for details). Taking this to your doctor and describing your symptoms may help.

With or without thyroid medication, there are certainly nutritional and lifestyle factors that will support your thyroid. Jump to Part 3 to find out more.

Fiona's story

Hashimoto's and gluten

Fiona is a 42-year-old accountant who called me one day feeling desperate. She had been diagnosed with hypothyroidism 10 years earlier, after the birth of her baby.

She had been taking thyroxine since then, and in the early days it had worked pretty well to combat her post-pregnancy fatigue, weight gain and low mood. However, in the past year or so, she had noticed her symptoms coming back. Her weight had crept up, she was increasingly exhausted and her mood was pretty low most of the time. She had gone to see her doctor who had told her she was fine and to up her dose a bit. It hadn't worked. So we started working together on why her thyroid might be struggling. When we got her tested it turned out she had raised antibodies indicating Hashimoto's disease, which is an autoimmune condition. Once we focused on the root cause of her immune overreaction, which ended up being a gluten sensitivity, she was able to dramatically improve her thyroid function. Here's what she said:

'I was so worried when my thyroid symptoms started coming back and all I could do was increase my medication. It felt like a stab in the dark. When I got tested, I was so relieved that we could go deeper and find out what was causing my condition rather than use the drugs as a sticking plaster. Once we found out it was gluten that was making my immune system attack my thyroid, it was a super easy fix. Learning how to cut gluten out of my life, whilst eating amazing food and not feeling deprived, was a huge relief to me. And the end result? Two stone lighter, loads more energy, and a happy balanced mood!'

SUMMARY

- Thyroid hormones are the switch on your metabolism – up or down
- Low thyroid is more common than high in women over 40
- Stress can crash your thyroid – you need to support your adrenals
- Symptoms can range vastly from fatigue and weight gain to depression and joint pain
- Your T4 hormone is the precursor to the active T3 – know your T3 levels
- Mainstream testing is often inadequate – get private tests if you are concerned
- Find the root cause of your low thyroid and you have a chance to reverse it

Quick tips

1. Fat is your friend – fats are the building blocks of hormones and cell membranes, so it's really important to include plenty of healthy fats in your diet.
2. Ditch the processed foods – cook from scratch wherever possible.
3. Up your protein – protein breaks down to amino acids, one of which is tyrosine, needed to make thyroid hormone.
4. Check your sugar intake – blood sugar balance is key, as too much insulin can suppress your thyroid. Avoid refined carbohydrates and sugar, and always try to eat protein and healthy fat with your food to slow the sugar release.
5. Avoid stimulants and artificial sweeteners – caffeine, sugar and alcohol increase insulin and cortisol and are not helping your thyroid. Artificial sweeteners are chemicals that can interfere with metabolism and damage your brain cells.
6. Eat five Brazil nuts each day – the selenium helps to make your thyroid work.
7. Ditch the gluten – try a few weeks without it to see if your symptoms improve.
8. Eat coconut oil – a saturated fat made of medium chain triglycerides, coconut oil helps to boost metabolism, helping your thyroid to do its job.
9. Check your iron levels – ask your doctor for a ferritin test. Low iron can cause low thyroid.
10. Get your sunshine! – vitamin D supports thyroid function – if you can't get enough sun exposure, take a D3 supplement.

4 – Oestrogen – your SEX hormone

Oestrogen (or more technically the three oestrogen hormones) is your main sex hormone and the one that gives you your feminine qualities and abilities – your curves, your breasts, your ability to have a baby, all due to oestrogen!

Whether you have children or not, from puberty to pregnancy to menopause, oestrogen has a huge impact on your life. As well as regulating your cycle, it also protects your bones, heart, muscle mass, brain and joints.

But it does have a less attractive side.

Over 80% of women experience symptoms due to the changes and fluctuations in their sex hormones and menstrual cycles between the ages of 40 and 55. And the changes in oestrogen levels can be particularly problematic.

After 40, your reproductive capability decreases. Your egg reserve, which started out as millions when you were born, dwindles down to the last few hundred during this time. You're coming to the end of your fertile years and, to add insult to injury, this transitional time can result in huge hormone fluctuations and debilitating symptoms.

'I'm too young for the menopause!' Many women don't realize their bodies are preparing for menopause – either they don't associate the symptoms (especially if they're not having hot flushes) or symptoms could be very similar to other hormone imbalances (such as hypothyroidism or adrenal stress).

Progesterone decline

Progesterone is the first hormone to decline as you age. As levels go down more quickly than oestrogen, the balance between the two can tip in oestrogen's favour – this is often referred to as oestrogen dominance. Progesterone is mainly produced after ovulation, so if you don't ovulate (which can happen frequently during perimenopause), production will be low and oestrogen will be dominant.

Progesterone helps prevent the uterine lining from getting too thick, so when levels are low, you can get heavy periods, PMS and cramping. It helps to calm oestrogen's stimulating effect in the brain by increasing a calming hormone called gamma-aminobutyric acid (GABA), so when there isn't enough progesterone, you can get increased anxiety and interrupted sleep.

High oestrogen (or too low progesterone)

Oestradiol is the strongest of the oestrogens we produce before menopause, and while essential in the right amounts for heart, brain, skin, bone and reproductive health, this is the hormone that is also growth promoting. It is there to help cells multiply in order to thicken the uterus wall to prepare for pregnancy. This is why too much of it can lead to proliferation of cancer cells.

When progesterone declines, you can have too much oestradiol and that can cause all sorts of symptoms, mainly relating to menstrual issues – heavy periods, bloating, lumpy or tender breasts, headaches, cramps, but longer term can lead to more serious conditions such as fibroids, cysts, endometriosis and breast and ovarian cancers.

Low oestrogen

Low levels of oestrogen, either due to fluctuations during perimenopause, or more permanent low levels post-menopause, can be equally damaging. Symptoms can include hot flushes, night sweats, vaginal dryness, depression, dry itchy skin, wrinkles, insomnia, brain fog and memory loss. Longer-term risks of more serious conditions include osteoporosis, heart disease and cognitive decline.

Don't forget testosterone!

Testosterone is often ignored in women, but it is vital for your health as you age. It is best known for its sex drive effects (for both men and women), but it also provides proteins needed for your heart, muscles and bones. Keeping up your muscle and bone strength is vital as you go through menopause to prevent osteoporosis. Testosterone is also needed for regulating blood sugar and insulin, and for brain health, keeping you focused, alert and happy.

Other factors

1. **Stress** – cortisol is our main stress hormone and when it's out of balance (high or low) it can dramatically affect the function of our other hormones. Cortisol is made from pregnenolone (the mother hormone) but so is progesterone. So when you're stressed, more cortisol is needed at the expense of progesterone, thereby increasing oestrogen dominance. Your adrenals are under even more pressure as they take over responsibility for producing your sex hormones when the ovaries decline. So if you are too stressed, they struggle to cope and sex hormone production is affected.

The sex hormone pathway

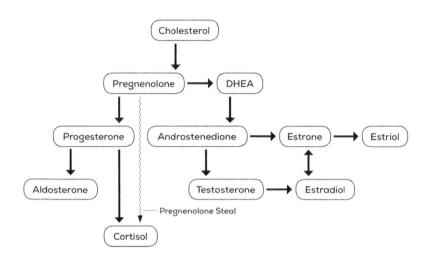

2. **Toxins** – our world is swimming in chemicals called 'xenoestrogens', so called because they are known to mimic our own natural oestrogen – artificially increasing our own oestrogen stores. Some of these include BPA (plastic bottles) and pesticides used on non-organic fruit and vegetables.
3. **Diet** – a high carb, sugar and processed food diet increases insulin levels. Insulin increases oestrogen production and also promotes inflammation, which is a further risk factor for chronic diseases such as diabetes, heart disease and cancer. Additionally, a diet lacking in good fats, protein, vitamins and minerals will affect hormone production, storage, transport and detoxification.
4. **Extra weight** – your fat cells cause oestrogen levels to rise as well, so the more fat you have, the more oestrogen you will make. This is not so bad when you are post-menopausal as the extra oestrogen is needed, but pre-menopause you don't need that extra supply.

5. **Birth control pills** can also lead to an excess of oestrogen – the pill suppresses ovulation to stop you getting pregnant. But this also reduces progesterone and adds to circulating oestrogen.
6. **Poor digestion or liver function** – can stop oestrogen being properly disposed of, and it can get recirculated, increasing the risk of oestrogen dominance.

Common symptoms

Low oestrogen

Hot flushes/night sweats – Oh the joy! Turning into a red-hot furnace without a moment's notice has to be the WORST hand dealt by Mother Nature. I have only had a few of these, but that was enough. There is nothing worse than internally combusting in the middle of a conversation or in a packed room, with sweat dripping off you and your make-up running down your face. You just have to get out of there fast. Some women have several of these a day, lasting from 30 seconds to five minutes or so. And then they continue through the night, waking you up in a pile of sweat, so now you can't sleep either! These hot flushes are still a bit of a mystery in the science world but are generally thought to be caused by low levels of oestrogen disturbing the temperature control centre of the brain (hypothalamus) and are made a lot worse by stress, anxiety, smoking, caffeine and alcohol.

Dryness – Oestrogen keeps your skin supple, soft and smooth. So when levels decline, we start to get itchy and dry skin, as well as wrinkles, crow's feet, age spots and pimples. Vaginal dryness (or the medical term – atrophic vaginitis!) is very common at this stage. Not only does your libido take a dive, but intercourse can also be difficult and painful.

Mood swings, crankiness – Oestrogen has a role in serotonin, GABA and dopamine production; the neurotransmitters that make you feel good. So when levels are too low, your feel-good factor goes missing. Stress has a hand in this too, as excess cortisol disturbs the normal biochemistry in the brain. It is also common to have feelings of depression at this time.

Weight gain – During the perimenopause years you might notice your weight creeping (or surging!) upwards, especially around the stomach and hips – the dreaded 'middle-age spread'. If your fluctuating oestrogen and cortisol are disturbing your brain biochemistry, you could be low on serotonin, which can result in craving carbohydrates. And when you are tired, moody and irritable all the time, you turn to sugar and processed carbs as your comfort food. Lack of sleep has also been linked to increased appetite.

Another theory of why women gain weight running up to the menopause is that as your ovarian function starts to decline, other sources of oestrogen production come into play. One of these alternative sources is fat cells. So sometimes your body will hang on to your fat stores so that it can get enough oestrogen produced, especially when you are under stress or on a poor diet.

Insomnia – Declining oestrogen and progesterone make it harder to get a good night's sleep, making you more tired and irritable during the day. Your sleep might also be interrupted by night sweats and having to change the bed sheets.

Memory loss/brain fog – Constantly losing things, forgetting people's names and struggling to remember what you did last week? Stopping in the middle of a sentence, losing your thread and finding it hard to concentrate? There are oestrogen receptors in the brain, and we know that oestrogen plays a role in brain cell health, memory, mood and thinking. Low testosterone can also contribute to a loss of mental agility.

Low libido/painful sex – To feel sexy you need good oestrogen levels (which is often why you are in the mood around the time of ovulation). If oestrogen is low, and you're feeling tired and irritable, it's going to be the last thing on your mind. Low testosterone will decrease your libido and low oestrogen can also be responsible for vaginal dryness, which is not going to help you feel sexy! And if you do manage to keep up your sex life, orgasms may be harder to achieve and less intense.

Joint pain and bone loss – Normal levels of oestrogen help to increase bone production and regulate fluid levels in your body, reducing inflammation and swelling around joints.

Irregular periods – Your ovaries are living out their usefulness. They are sputtering out the last few eggs in a very ad hoc way, sometimes not managing to ovulate at all, sometimes with wayward timing. This is totally normal, however hugely inconvenient for us women! Not knowing when your period will come, having two- or 10-day bleeds, sometimes gushing sometimes trickling, odd spotting in between, you just want it to be over!

High oestrogen (or too low progesterone)

PMS – Painful cramps like you had when you were a teenager? You thought you were past all that PMS stuff and now it's worse than ever. If you have any of these symptoms, it's worth checking in with your doctor – heavy periods or cramps can be an indicator of something more serious.

Breast tenderness – High oestrogen or low progesterone can often result in painful breasts, especially during the luteal period of your cycle (up to two weeks before your period).

Bloating/water retention – High oestrogen levels encourage fluid retention and bloating, especially around the ankles and tummy area.

Headaches or migraines – Usually around ovulation or just before your period, headaches can result from a surge in oestrogen and not enough progesterone to balance it. Oestrogen dilates blood vessels, and this can result in a build-up of fluid and pressure in the brain.

Fibroids, cysts, endometriosis, PCOS – These conditions can be driven by excess oestrogen (and androgen) levels (see Chapter 1).

If your symptoms are having a big impact on your life or you are in premature menopause, you should seek medical advice. Don't get caught up in the 'menopause is natural so put up with it' brigade if you are suffering. There is no question about giving insulin to diabetic patients, or thyroxine for those with hypothyroidism – so sex hormone replacement should also be an option for anyone. But the important thing is that you make an informed choice, and choose the best path for you.

The standard medical treatment is HRT – hormone replacement therapy. This is usually a mix of synthetic oestrogen and progestin (an artificial progesterone). There are other forms and some doctors do prescribe bio-identical hormones, a more natural alternative (more on that in Chapter 12).

There are many ways to support this time of your life naturally. Balancing your hormone health through food, lifestyle choices and targeted supplements can make a huge difference.

Jump to Part 3 to find out how you can do that.

Polly's story

Hot flush hell

Polly is a 50-year-old office manager, who was suffering terribly with hot flushes and night sweats. It was getting to be so embarrassing when she had an episode during the day, as there was no warning. It could happen in the middle of a meeting or on a crowded train on the way to work. The heat would start to rise from her legs and when it hit her head she would instantly start sweating. And during the night she would wake up in a pile of sweat and have to change the sheets. She was exhausted! She had been offered HRT, but wanted to see if she could treat it naturally. We started her on a hormone-balancing programme with plenty of phytoestrogens (flaxseeds, lentils, chickpeas) plus some targeted supplements to boost her hormones.

Here's what she said:
'Hot flushes were ruining my life! I was having over 10 a day, and they would happen any time, any place. I had to carry a small towel with me, plus a mini fan, and just hoped there was somewhere to hide whenever it happened. I was so tired as well, as the night sweats would interrupt my sleep. When I started eating to balance my oestrogen, things started to improve. Then we looked at possible triggers for the sweats. Stress was a big one, so I started some deep breathing exercises every day, and that really helped. I also realized that alcohol was a big trigger. After two weeks alcohol-free on the programme, my hot flushes had reduced by half. By putting all these things in place, I am now sweat-free and feeling confident again!'

SUMMARY

- Oestrogen and progesterone start to decline from the age of 35 as your egg reserve begins to run out
- Progesterone declines more rapidly than oestrogen, which can tip you into oestrogen dominance
- Oestrogen can fluctuate wildly during perimenopause, so you can experience symptoms of high and low oestrogen
- Testosterone is also important – it's another hormone that declines as you get older
- HRT is not the only option available

Quick tips

1. **Eat your broccoli** – cruciferous veg (e.g. broccoli, cabbage, cauliflower, watercress, kale, rocket, Brussels sprouts) can really help your liver with detoxification of oestrogen.
2. **Ditch the sugar** – choose a low GL diet with limited sugar and carbs. Stay away from artificial sugars though (now known to make you gain weight!). This will help balance your blood sugar and reduce insulin levels.
3. **Sprinkle those seeds** – flaxseeds, chia, pumpkin, sesame and sunflower seeds all contain good amounts of protein, vitamins, minerals, fibre and phytoestrogens that can help to regulate oestrogen levels. Sprinkle in smoothies, yoghurt, porridge, salads.
4. **Get pooping!** – improve your digestion so you can eliminate excess oestrogen – increase your fibre (wholegrains, fruit, veg, nuts, seeds) and probiotic foods (live natural yoghurt, sauerkraut, kefir, miso).

Avoid wheat and dairy if you suspect any intolerances (bloating, gas, cramps).

5. **Avoid chemical oestrogens** – swap your plastic for glass, stainless steel or ceramic.

6. **Switch to natural brands for your toiletries, cosmetics and household products.**

7. **Go organic** – limit your exposure to pesticides. Especially important for those fruit and veg where you are eating the skins (apples, berries, peppers, etc).

8. **Lose weight** – if you do all the above you will lose weight naturally – less fat, less oestrogen production.

9. **Reduce your stress** – schedule in some relaxation every day, even if it's just 10 minutes of deep breathing. This will help balance your cortisol.

10. **Limit alcohol and caffeine** – this can help reduce hot flushes and blood sugar imbalances.

11. **Consider more natural methods of contraception and/ or hormone replacement** – there are plenty of choices now for contraception. If you've been on the pill, implant or Mirena coil for a long time, consider switching. You can also swap from HRT to body-identical HRT, a more natural alternative (see Chapter 12).

PART 2

WHY YOUR HORMONES NEED HELP

CHAPTER 4

THE BIG DIETARY AND LIFESTYLE SABOTEURS

Your Feisty 4 hormones are incredibly sensitive things! They react very quickly (and sometimes dramatically) to outside influences on a daily basis – what nutrients they are getting, what stress levels they are being exposed to, what environmental toxins they encounter and what kind of movement the body is going through.

The good news is that if you're doing the right things, your hormones can rebalance quickly. Here are the top four dietary and lifestyle hormone saboteurs that you need to be aware of.

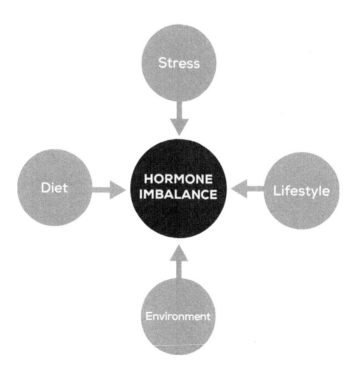

<u>Grab your workbook and tick off the things that you are doing that you think may be affecting your hormones.</u>

Diet

Your diet is number one for a reason. Hormones need a steady stream of nutrients for them to work efficiently. Do they get what they need? Often not in our modern diet.

Many women are eating the wrong foods and not supplying their hormones with the building blocks they need to work properly. You need adequate protein to produce and transport hormones, vitamins and minerals to help them metabolize and break down, good fats to help them work, antioxidants and phytonutrients to protect them, good carbohydrates, fibre and plenty of clean water to help them move around and detoxify.

Our typical diets can be missing plenty of these nutrients (not enough vegetables, protein, good fats, water), but even if you are eating the best diet possible, you can have problems digesting and absorbing the nutrients from your food due to an imbalance in gut bacteria or inflammation in your digestive tract (see Chapter 6 for more on the gut).

Without the right nutrients you start getting symptoms of hormone imbalance (fatigue, weight gain, sluggishness etc) and our natural instinct is to go for a fast fix with the wrong foods (carbs, sugar, bad fats), making our symptoms even worse.

How does your diet affect your Feisty 4 hormones?

1. Your diet and cortisol
What you eat (or don't eat) can be a stress on the body, and when the body is stressed, you get a cortisol release. And if this is

happening day in, day out, all that cortisol is going to take a toll on your weight, energy levels, mood, brain and general well-being. What foods are likely to be potential stressors? Processed foods, sugar, refined carbs, vegetable oils, food chemicals, alcohol, caffeine and foods that you may be sensitive to.

2. Your diet and insulin

The wrong foods can spike your blood sugar and make you overproduce insulin, your fat-storing hormone. And as we have already seen, too much insulin not only puts more fat down, but it also increases your risk of further complications such as diabetes, dementia and heart disease.

3. Your diet and thyroid

The wrong food choices can prevent your thyroid from getting the nutrients it needs to work well – slowing down your metabolism and putting you into sluggish, fat-storing mode.

4. Your diet and oestrogen

If you haven't got enough protein, healthy fat or nutrients in your diet, then your sex hormone production will be affected, putting your body under more stress as it tries to rebalance everything.

Convenience and big bucks

Unfortunately, with our modern-day western diet and fast-paced lifestyle – the food industry has taken advantage of us...

They have manufactured fast and easy foods that are perfect for our busy lifestyles; ready meals, prepared sauces, packets and tubs of all things easy and quick. It has turned food into a convenience rather than a pleasure. And it has helped to produce a whole generation of people that can't (and won't) cook from scratch.

For me this is a tragedy, and we are going to see the consequences of it in the future. A recent survey suggested 33% of 24–35 year olds couldn't boil an egg! A generation of adults consuming convenience foods, and no cooking skills to pass down to the kids. It's a downward spiral unless we can re-educate people about the benefits of fresh real food!

The problem with these processed convenience foods is that they are made on the cheap, with absolutely no thought to your health and every thought to company profit. They want you to come back for more of course.

Here's what's in most processed and packaged foods:

A tablespoon of trans-fats
These 'fake' foods are made using cheap industrial vegetable oils, which do the job to cook the food but they are no good for your health. These volatile plant oils go rancid on heating and processing, turning into trans-fats that the body has no idea what to do with and treats as toxic waste!

Don't be fooled by the term 'vegetable oil' – they are nothing to do with vegetables and are definitely not wanted in your five a day! Check out Chapter 5 for the truth about fat.

Spoonfuls of sugar
The next ingredient is sugar, which of course is added in spoonfuls to make the food taste good (who doesn't like sugar?). And we know that fat and sugar together bring out the addict in you (the combination lights up your dopamine receptors) and does nothing for your blood sugar balance (increased insulin = increased fat stores!) – think doughnut as the perfect example. I like to call it 'sweet fat'.

A handful of salt

Then they shove in some processed table salt to stimulate your taste buds even more, which of course increases your blood pressure and puts your electrolyte balance out (stressing your body!) and dehydrating your cells.

A cup full of chemicals

And of course they want their products to look good, have the right texture and last a while on the shelf, so they add a whole bunch of additives, colours, flavourings and preservatives.

And then they often market it as a health product! One of the worst ready meals I have found came from a leading weight-loss company!

We are so used to seeing these products in stores, on TV and in everyone else's shopping baskets, that we are treating these 'fake' foods as totally normal and safe.

When you eat these foods, you are getting very few nutrients and a ton of stuff the body doesn't recognize. This is a huge stress on the body, and we know what cortisol likes to do, don't we?

We have a food industry that is not interested in health. And a health industry that's not interested in food!

Let's get away from fake processed foods and back to foods the body was designed to eat. See Chapter 7, Step 1 for more.

Stress

You learnt in Chapter 2 how cortisol is released when you are stressed, and how it can make you fat, tired and downright miserable. Too much cortisol also uses up many of your nutrient stores. It rapidly depletes B vitamins and vitamin C, as well as magnesium, all nutrients required for good hormone function and energy production. Which is why stress can be so exhausting!

Stress also suppresses your digestive function, often resulting in IBS-like symptoms and undigested food. This can damage your gut lining, and upset the delicate balance of gut bacteria, putting you at increased risk of infection and autoimmune reactions. See Chapter 6 on how your gut and hormones are linked.

As you head towards menopause, the adrenal glands take over the production of sex hormones from the ovaries. If your adrenals are struggling to cope due to high stress demands, supply of sex hormones can suffer. This is why perimenopausal and post-menopausal symptoms can include brain fog, memory loss, low libido, vaginal dryness and hot flushes.

How does stress affect your Feisty 4 hormones?

1. Stress and cortisol
Cortisol gets released when a stress gets triggered. And it stays high when your source of stress doesn't go away. And high cortisol contributes to belly fat, fatigue, anxiety, sugar cravings, brain fog, mood swings, PMS, infertility and a whole lot more!

2. Stress and insulin
Cortisol's job is to put sugar into your blood (so you can 'fight or flight'). Whenever you have sugar in your blood, insulin has to be released to mop it up and take it to your cells. The trouble is that if you're stressed all the time and there's plenty of cortisol around, then you're going to need lots of insulin too. That puts you on the blood sugar roller coaster that we talked about in Chapter 3, triggering those blood sugar lows that can result in energy dips, cravings, mood swings, brain fog and poor sleep.

3. Stress and thyroid

I talked about cortisol in Chapter 3 having a dominant effect over all your other hormones, including your thyroid. You need cortisol for your thyroid to work properly – it helps convert your thyroid hormones into their active form. When there's too much or too little cortisol it can affect this conversion rate – it makes sense for the body to conserve your energy when you're in survival mode. It does that by suppressing your thyroid, therefore reducing your metabolism (and stopping your body burning fat!).

4. Stress and oestrogen

Stress and cortisol also suppress all your sex hormones. If your body is in survival mode, the last thing it's worrying about is your reproductive system or whether you feel sexy or not! So when you are stressed for long periods of time, it can result in PMS, heavy periods, irregular periods, anxiety, mood swings, infertility and of course low sex drive.

Are you a stress junkie?

Do you measure your importance, value or success in life based on how busy you are? How full your calendar is? Does it make you feel like your life is more successful the more hectic you are? Being 'stressed' or crazy busy these days can look like a measure of how important you feel. Here are some clues to tell if you might be addicted to stress:

- You're a Type A personality and thrive under pressure; you get bored sitting still and who needs sleep anyway?
- You're wired, and know you need to switch off, but can't relax whatever you do.
- You pride yourself on how busy you are, you're 'crazy busy' you tell your friends, like it makes you more important. Your to-do list is like a badge of honour!

- You're addicted to drama. Your life is like a soap opera.
- You're terrified of missing out – you'll check your phone even in the best situations.
- You're addicted to the quiet drama of constant anxiety and worry.

Cortisol has been shown to light up your dopamine receptors in the brain, just like crack cocaine! And when you're exposed daily to stressful situations, your brain can get hooked on that euphoric feeling, and boom, you're a STRESSAHOLIC.

Just like drugs and alcohol, stress can be an avoidance tactic. A way to distract you from the real world and your real problems, says Debbie Mandel, author of *Addicted to Stress*.

And it's insidious in our modern-day society. We are all bombarded by 'stuff' that keeps us addicted: 24-hour news, video games, instant messaging, never-ending emails, online shopping! We don't get a chance to stop and breathe!

Social media is one of the biggest addictions going. I have to limit my Facebook time otherwise I can waste hours lost in my newsfeed. Corporates are investing big in 'digital detoxes' for employees to get them more focused on the job.

And you only have to look at the kids to know where it's all going. Their smartphones are literally an extension of their physical bodies! No wonder we have a generation of stressed-out kids. We have to show them how to switch off or we'll be generating a whole new set of stress junkies.

Wake up!

Stress is not cool. It's not a measure of how important your life is. You're not going to feel that important when you're seriously ill, or even dead. Harsh, yes, but reducing stress is that important; it's not only making you fat, cranky, forgetful, exhausted, a sugar junkie, and unsexy, it's also a ticking time bomb. Let's wake up, not just for our own sake, but for all the people who depend on us!

Stressed, me?

When I was studying nutrition at college in my mid 40s, we were offered a free stress test by one of the labs. I was reluctant to do it at the time, thinking it was a waste of time. I wasn't a 'stressy' person at all, there was no way it was going to be an issue.

So blow me down when the test results showed I had adrenal fatigue! But looking back, two emergency C-sections in my 30s on top of raising kids for the last 10 years – that will put a strain on anyone's adrenal reserves.

I was surprised because I didn't feel my life was particularly stressful. I am lucky to have a very happy marriage and a loving family network. Many people have a much bigger stress load to deal with. It just shows you how a fairly 'normal' lifestyle can affect you (even if you think you're pretty laid-back and have everything under control!).

You certainly don't need to have had kids either to suffer from stress or other hormonal imbalances. Many women in their 40s struggle with the same issues, children or not. We all have our sources of stress (sometimes it's internal and we are unaware of it), and perimenopause happens to each of us!

Sleep

And are you sleeping well? Chris Kresser, a respected naturopath in the US, writes about the importance of sleep and says:

'You can eat a perfect diet and take all the right supplements, but if you're not sleeping well and managing your stress, all bets are off...'

So many women are suffering from insomnia. I guess it's not surprising if we are all stressed. Getting to sleep, staying asleep and waking up refreshed is seemingly rare these days.

A GMTV poll in 2006 reported that '42% of people in the South East sleep for less than 5 hours a night' and more than 10 million prescriptions for sleeping pills are handed out each year. That's incredible isn't it?

Insomniacs have been shown to have higher cortisol levels. And the higher your cortisol, the harder it is to get a good night's sleep! And if you're sleep deprived, it takes much longer to clear cortisol from your system.

Sleep is so important – it's when the body restores energy levels and repairs any damage done. It resets your metabolism and sets you up for the next day – we all know how debilitating a bad night's sleep can be (any new parent can vouch for that!).

Why is sleep good for you?

- It keeps you YOUNG – lack of sleep can not only make you look older, but it can age you on the inside too
- It keeps you HAPPY – how grumpy do you feel when you haven't slept well? Studies show you feel less empathy for others and you are much more likely to have arguments with loved ones
- It gives you ENERGY – obvious one, but so many women are TATT (tired all the time) and it's not rocket science – they need more sleep!

- It helps with your MEMORY – deep sleep is when the brain consolidates everything it has learnt from the day and stores it away as a memory. Lack of sleep interferes with this, so you can be increasingly forgetful (that's why it's not a good idea to do an all-nighter cramming for exams!)
- It helps to keep your weight under control – lack of sleep slows down your metabolism, increases cortisol and insulin (which likes to put fat on around your middle), reduces thyroid hormones (responsible for fat burning) and increases hunger hormones
- It helps prevent Alzheimer's and dementia – recent studies indicate that the brain performs a kind of 'detoxifying wash' during your deep sleep, clearing out waste and amyloid plaques (risk factors for Alzheimer's)

There is now overwhelming evidence that sleep deprivation has a massive effect on your health, and chronic lack of sleep has a cumulative effect (you can't get your missed sleep back)!

For many people, sleeping well gets harder as you get older. There are several reasons for this:

- **Stress** – cortisol is supposed to drop at night, so that your body can relax and sleep. If you have excess cortisol running around your system, you are on alert and can't relax. This can happen when you stay up late to work, surf the net or watch TV.
- **Blood sugar imbalance** – this is often the case when you have no trouble falling asleep but wake up during the night and can't get back to sleep. Low blood sugar during the night caused by eating too many refined carbs and sugar or alcohol, can wake you up – it's a stressor on the body. Balancing your blood sugar levels during the day can really help with good quality sleep.

- **Too many stimulants** – coffee, tea, chocolate, energy and fizzy drinks and alcohol can all affect your sleep pattern. We all know those people who can drink coffee all day and sleep like a baby, but we all have a genetic capability to detoxify caffeine and alcohol, and for some of us it takes a long time to rid it from our system. Stimulants can also disrupt the production of serotonin, which makes melatonin.

- **Lack of melatonin** (the sleep hormone) – stress, a disrupted circadian rhythm (e.g. shift work) and artificial light can all disrupt melatonin production. You have light sensors all over your body that tell your brain when it is dark and time to go to sleep. Any source of light at night (such as computer lights, streetlights, alarm clocks and mobile phones) can disturb these messages and therefore your melatonin production. And melatonin is a potent antioxidant and tumour suppressor. Which means as well as a bad night's sleep, you might be increasing your risk of chronic disease if your melatonin production is compromised.

- **Bedroom environment** – if your room is too warm it can interfere with your body temperature and stop you sleeping.

- **Lack of thyroid hormone** – can reduce the amount of deep sleep you're getting. Low thyroid symptoms can include waking up unrefreshed, with a puffy face and/ or eyes. And sleep deprivation lowers thyroid hormone – a vicious cycle.

- **Progesterone** – aids sleep, so if you are low (which is the case for many women over 40!) it may affect your sleep.

As well as having too much light at night interfering with your natural sleep pattern, you may also be keeping yourself awake artificially, with too much screen time just before bed. The blue light from most electronic devices has a particular stimulatory effect. How do you expect to wind down if you are checking Facebook and emails? Your brain needs to slow down before making you feel sleepy. Even watching the news before bed can overexcite your brain and keep you awake.

How much sleep do you need?

You sleep in cycles from wakefulness to REM to non-REM deep sleep. Each cycle lasts approximately 1.5 hours and most of us need at least five cycles to feel fully rested. That's around 7.5 hours, but of course everyone is different and this may vary. A good test is to count back from when you wake up naturally (with no alarm). So if you need to get up at 6am every day, try going to bed earlier and earlier until you can wake up naturally. It may need some experimentation, but this is a good way to know for sure how much your body needs. (My bedtime to wake up naturally at 6am is 10pm, so I need eight hours sleep).

Are you staying up too late?

You might have heard that the hours before midnight are more restorative? There is some truth in that. From around 11pm til 3am, you have more deep non-REM sleep. After 3am, the balance changes and you have more REM sleep (the stage associated with dreaming).

The deep non-REM sleep is when the body stores and consolidates its learning and memory, and repairs and regenerates cells and tissues, so this deep sleep is what you're aiming for. Therefore, staying up past midnight when you're getting up early is putting you at a huge disadvantage!

Your diet and lifestyle can make everything worse. Too much caffeine, alcohol and carbohydrates can stop you getting a good night's sleep. Lack of sleep is a stress on the body, which raises your cortisol levels, which disturbs your sleep – a vicious hormonal cycle.

Jump to Chapter 7, Step 2 of the Happy Hormone Code for how to improve your stress and sleep.

Environment

Our lives today are much more toxic than ever before. With modern technology, we have devised a huge number of new chemicals that we were never exposed to previously. According to the US Environmental Protection Agency, there are more than 84,000 chemical substances listed on their inventory (and rising!).

We all want to look and smell nice. We all want our homes to be clean and our furniture to be flameproof. We like our gardens to be weed-free, and our pets to be flea-free. We need to wear sunscreen and we like our food to not stick to the pan. We want our hard-to-wash clothes to be clean and our hair to be coloured, permed or straightened.

All of this though might come at a cost. There's no absolute proof that each chemical is dangerous, but there is plenty of concern amongst the scientific and medical world.

Individual chemicals are pronounced 'safe' by the authorities and are used liberally. However, what we don't know is the cumulative effect of so many chemicals in our system. This 'chemical soup' is a new and unknown quantity, and nobody really knows what it's doing to us, or our hormone function. These chemicals are treated as 'innocent until proven guilty', but shouldn't it be the opposite? Guilty until proven innocent? I for one would feel a lot safer!

In 2005, the EWG (Environmental Working Group) in the US identified 167 synthetic chemicals and carcinogens in the bodies of the average US citizen! Particular concerns are for unborn babies and young children as they are more vulnerable to some of these toxins.

Women are also more vulnerable – it is thought that female livers have less capacity for detoxification of toxins due to the fact that we have so much oestrogen to deal with. Plus of course we are likely to use more personal care products than most men.

The World Health Organization produced a report in 2012 pressing for more research but this will take time, so it's up to us to protect ourselves, and the next generations, as much as we can.

> *'Close to 800 chemicals are known or suspected to be capable of interfering with hormones… The vast majority have not been tested at all.'*
>
> *WHO 2012*

And as many of these toxins are fat soluble, it might not be surprising that they end up in your fat cells and in your brain. Toxic exposure has been linked to weight gain and neurological conditions such as depression, Parkinson's and Alzheimer's.

Endocrine Disrupting Chemicals (EDCs)

What we do know is that certain chemicals have been shown to act as Endocrine Disrupting Chemicals or EDCs. That is, they are molecularly similar to certain hormones, and your body finds it hard to distinguish between the fake and the real. Your genes play a huge part in how well you detoxify chemicals and some people can tolerate a huge number of toxins with no apparent effects. However, for many of us, these chemicals can cause huge hormonal disruption.

A scientific statement issued by the US Endocrine Society in 2009 expressed concern about EDCs and the grave health issues they can cause, including cancer, heart disease, diabetes, PCOS, obesity, thyroid disease and reproductive issues.

An excerpt from the report regarding EDCs:

> 'Even infinitesimally low levels of exposure – indeed, any level of exposure at all – may cause endocrine or reproductive abnormalities, particularly if exposure occurs during a critical developmental window. Surprisingly, low doses may even exert more potent effects than higher doses… There is no endocrine system that is immune to these substances, because of the shared properties of the chemicals and the similarities of the receptors and enzymes involved in the synthesis, release, and degradation of hormones.'

Eek! This is scary stuff, as we have no idea what the longer term effects are of all these chemicals.

> 'The diverse systems affected by EDCs likely include all hormonal systems… Effects can lead to obesity, infertility, learning difficulties, diabetes, heart disease and others.'
>
> WHO 2012

How do these EDCs affect your Feisty 4 hormones?

1. Chemicals and cortisol
Toxins are a stress on the body – and when the body feels threatened it stimulates the release of cortisol to keep it safe. We've heard how too much cortisol affects all your other hormones and can cause all sorts of symptoms.

2. Chemicals and insulin

Studies have shown that exposure to EDCs can damage the cells in your pancreas that produce insulin, and actually disrupt the action of insulin itself, making your body more prone to storing fat instead of burning it, and increasing the risk of diabetes.

3. Chemicals and thyroid

EDCs have been shown to impair your thyroid hormones – making your metabolism slow and therefore contributing to weight gain, fatigue, brain fog, anxiety, hair loss, digestive issues and many more.

4. Chemicals and oestrogen

Many of these EDCs contain 'fake' oestrogens that act like your own oestrogen, attaching to your cell receptors and causing disruption. Studies have linked EDCs with all sorts of hormone conditions such as early puberty, infertility, endometriosis, miscarriage and oestrogen-driven cancers.

How toxic are you?

Let's have a look at the average working woman's daily routine:

She wakes up and has a shower: shampoo, conditioner, shower gel, shower curtain
She towels herself dry and puts on: talc, body lotion, deodorant
She brushes her teeth with toothpaste and maybe uses some mouthwash
She does her face: moisturizer, make-up
She does her hair: hair products, hairspray
She might do her nails: nail varnish, nail varnish remover
She puts on some perfume and she's ready!

That's potentially over 14 different products before she does anything else! Just have a look at the ingredients label on any of these products and you will see how many chemicals each one has, and you will see how the average exposure is estimated at over 500 chemicals just in the morning routine.

As she leaves the house, she drives or walks to work. She is exposed to car fumes and pollution.

During the day, she may come into contact with any of these products:

Sun cream
Tampons
Cleaning products
Laundry products
Antibacterial soap
New furniture
New carpet
Paint
Air fresheners
Candles
Cooking pans
Plastic wrap
Plastic bottles
Tupperware
Aluminium foil
Hairdresser – colouring, treatments
Nail salon
Dry cleaners
Factory fumes
Aeroplane cabin air
Food additives and pesticides
Tap water
Cigarette smoke
Charred food

All these products contain some form of toxin for the body to deal with. It can put a real strain on your liver, which can struggle to cope with the onslaught! When that happens, toxins can recirculate and accumulate.

Are toxins making you fat?

A new group of toxins has been labelled 'obesogens'. These are chemicals known to promote obesity and fat storage. According to Stephen Perrine, author of *The New American Diet*, chemical obesogens can trick the body into responding inappropriately, and are able to stimulate and inhibit hormone production and function.

Not only are these toxins causing fat gain, but they could also be preventing fat loss. To protect you from the harmful effects of toxins, the body stores them away in your fat cells. Most toxins are 'lipophilic' meaning they are attracted to fat, so this is a good place for them to live. Unfortunately, this means that the more fat you have, the more potential toxins you are storing.

If you start to lose fat, these toxins can be released into your body to travel around and cause havoc. This is common during or after a detox programme, often experienced as headaches, fatigue, joint pain and generally feeling rotten.

Toxins can damage your cell membranes and hormone receptors, making it difficult for hormones to enter the cell and do their thing. They can also damage your mitochondria (the little batteries inside every cell) so that they can't produce enough energy, making you feel tired. And once inside your cells they can alter your DNA and affect your gene expression, making you much more susceptible to disease.

SO, if you are doing any kind of detox programme, it is really important to support your liver and digestion so that you can eliminate the freed-up toxins from your system.

What are these toxins?

Here is a selection of the chemicals we know about:

BPA

Bisphenol A is the best known and the most widely studied EDC in terms of research. The list of its damaging effects grows by the day as more research emerges. So far we have links with obesity, diabetes, thyroid disease, breast and prostate cancer, brain tumours, reproductive disorders, asthma, heart disease, liver damage and neurological conditions. Eek!

This plastic is everywhere and a study in 2008 showed that 92% of the US population had BPA in their blood. More worryingly, BPA has been found in pregnant women and umbilical cords. It was only in 2011 that BPA was banned in baby bottles in Europe, but at the time of writing, the US still allows it!

Most exposure is from drinking water out of plastic bottles (one study found that you can substantially increase your BPA levels after only a week of drinking from plastic water bottles!). BPA is also found in hard plastic containers, plastic wrap and drinks bottles with the number 7 on the base. And in the lining of canned foods. Watch out for tinned tomatoes – the acidity of the tomatoes can cause the BPA to leach from the can lining into the food.

It is also found in till receipts and dental composites (those white fillings that are meant to be better than amalgams!).

Phthalates

These are synthetic chemicals added to plastics to make them flexible. Anything with PVC has phthalates in it – cling film, vinyl shower curtains, shiny raincoats, plastic toys. Even that 'new car' smell – that's phthalates in the air.

They are also found in anything with 'fragrance' or 'parfum' listed in the ingredients – scented candles, cosmetics, perfumes, shampoo, lotions, air fresheners, cleaning materials.

Phthalates are particularly dangerous in pregnancy and have been linked to genital defects and obesity in children. There are also links to diabetes and insulin resistance.

Petrochemicals

Benzene and benzoates are found in exhaust fumes, petrol, cosmetics, oils, fragrances. They mainly affect the respiratory system.

Pesticides

Found in non-organic food produce, insect repellent sprays (DEET), weedkillers. They are designed to kill living organisms such as plants, bacteria, insects and fungi. Imagine what they are doing to your friendly gut bacteria and immune system? And because they are fat soluble, they are stored in your fat cells, potentially messing up your metabolism.

These chemicals have been strongly linked with increased risk of many chronic diseases including neurological conditions, diabetes, obesity, cancer and hormone imbalances.

PFCs (perfluorinated chemicals)

Mostly found in non-stick cookware (e.g. Teflon), food packaging, stain and water repellents (e.g. Scotchgard and

Gore-Tex). If you boil water in a Teflon pan, you'll be able to taste the chemical – and that's leaching into your food every time you cook. PFCs have been found to be toxic to the brain, and are associated with increased insulin resistance.

Flame retardants

PBDEs (polybrominated diphenyl ethers) are everywhere! In your mattress, carpet, furniture, electrical appliances, computers, baby equipment, paint – and they get into house dust, which we inhale.

Fluoride

Fluoride competes (and wins!) with iodine and can stop it making thyroid hormones. It can also interfere with the pineal gland, which makes melatonin.

This stuff is in our toothpaste and in some water supplies. I would recommend you do your own research on this one as it's a hot topic! But in my view it is well worth avoiding. You can buy fluoride-free toothpaste (my 14-year-old daughter has never had fluoride in her life and her teeth are perfect) and you can filter your water if it has been added.

Chlorine

A gas from the same 'halogen' group of chemicals as fluoride, best known as the cleaning agent in swimming pools, it can also displace iodine in the thyroid gland and mimic oestrogen.

It is also in tap water, bleach and disinfectant, and we are particularly vulnerable in the shower, as the chlorine gas escapes from the water and we inhale it.

Beauty products

We are slowly waking up to the harsh chemicals we put on our bodies every day.

Your skin is the largest organ in your body. While it protects you from the outside (bacteria, temperature, water, etc), it is super-absorbent. In less than a minute, what you put on your skin is absorbed into your bloodstream. This is handy for hormone creams or nicotine patches, but not so good for toxic chemicals!

If you eat something toxic, it has a hard time surviving. It has to get through stomach acid, then your immune system in your gut; it's a good defence against toxins that you ingest. You don't have that defence for toxins you put on your skin. They go straight into your bloodstream.

Here are the top 10 chemicals to avoid in your personal products:

1. Parabens – found in cosmetics, skincare, fake-tanning lotion
2. DEA (diethanolamine), MEA (monoethanolamine), TEA (methylamine) – lathering agent in shampoo, conditioner, lotions
3. Sodium laureth (or lauryl) sulphate (SLS, SLES) – in shampoo, conditioner
4. Polyethylene glycol (PEG), propylene glycol or isopropyl alcohol (aka antifreeze!) – found in many shampoos, skincare products
5. Ammonium xylenesulfonate and formaldehyde – found in nail polish
6. Aluminium chloride – found in anti-perspirants (also butane and propane in spray anti-perspirants)
7. Octinoxate – found in sun cream, hair dye, nail varnish, lipstick, skin creams
8. PABA – in sun cream

9. BHA (butylated hydroxyanisole) and BHT (butylated hydroxytoluene) – preservatives found in many skincare products
10. Phthalates – found in perfume, candles, air fresheners, cleaning products and anything with 'fragrance' in the ingredients

Download the App 'Think Dirty' to check how clean some of your favourite products are.

There are many more that are not listed here. My ultimate rule is:

<u>If it's something you wouldn't put in your mouth, don't put it on your skin!</u>

Medications

Medications are designed to help you fight disease and manage symptoms. But they are foreign compounds that also need to be detoxified by the liver. Like toxins, some of them can mess with your hormones, cause side effects and longer-term risks. A few examples are:

- Oral contraceptive pill (or birth control pill) – containing synthetic hormones that are designed to prevent ovulation (and therefore pregnancy). They can have a significant number of potential side effects, including nausea, weight gain, headaches, mood swings and low libido, as well as an increased risk of thrombosis and breast cancer.
- HRT – synthetic (not body identical) hormone replacement – long-term use can increase the risk of stroke, heart disease and breast, ovarian and uterine cancers.
- Steroids – side effects can include fatigue, high blood pressure, weight gain, mood swings, digestive issues,

low immunity, high blood sugar, muscle weakness and thinning bones.

- Antacids or PPIs – designed to suppress stomach acid production, these medications can impair digestion and absorption of nutrients and reduce immune function.
- Antidepressants – designed (for short-term use only) to increase serotonin, side effects can include anxiety, digestive issues, sweating, palpitations, fatigue, poor sleep, headaches, low sex drive and dizziness.
- Painkillers – NSAIDs (nonsteroidal anti-inflammatory drugs) like ibuprofen and aspirin can have many potential side effects including damage to the gut lining, impaired absorption of nutrients and leakage of waste and toxins into the bloodstream.

Many drugs can deplete the body of essential nutrients, in particular B vitamins, magnesium and zinc – all required for energy and hormone production, as well as liver detoxification pathways. A great book to read on this is *Drug Muggers* by Suzy Cohen.

What's in the water?

Our water supply is supposed to be 'clean', and compared to the developing world, it probably is. How sure are you of what's in it though? Many people drink tap water with no problem, however I am not so trusting. Contaminants such as fluoride, chlorine, lead and aluminium are often found in general water supplies and can interfere with hormone function.

Smoking

Cigarette smoke is obviously toxic and we know about the lung cancer risk. But it also affects your hormones. It can reduce oestrogen levels and bring on early menopause. It can also cause infertility. Women who smoke are at higher risk of diabetes and osteoporosis. Smoking stimulates free radical production, increasing wrinkles and killing off cells. At the same time, it depletes vitamin C, which attacks free radicals! Cigarettes contain over 4000 compounds, including nicotine, carbon monoxide, lead, ammonia, hydrogen cyanide and cadmium. Cadmium is a heavy metal that can stay in the body for years. It inhibits the utilization of zinc, an essential mineral for hormones and fertility. If you can't give up, make sure you are supplementing plenty of vitamin C, zinc and antioxidants.

Step 3 of the Happy Hormone Code in Chapter 7 will show you how to clean up your environment and minimize exposure to toxins.

Lifestyle

Physical activity

We all need it, about 30% of the world doesn't get any, and some of us do too much. Exercise is vital for hormone balance, as not only does it help get nutrients around the body but it also has been shown to reduce stress levels and also increase your insulin function.

> Katy Bowman, author of *Move Your DNA*, says:
> *'You can eat the perfect diet, sleep eight hours a night, and use only baking soda and vinegar to clean your house, but without the loads created by natural movement, all of these worthy efforts are thwarted at a cellular level, and your optimal wellness level remains elusive.'*

But there are a lot of myths out there about exercise. Especially for women over 40.

We are constantly told to **eat less and move more** – calories in, calories out right? Burn baby burn!

For a start, this message is not the right message for women over 40 who have raging hormones to consider (see Chapter 5) – but the assumption is that it's a general message that is true for everyone. SO you join a gym or start running, or even sign up to the latest 'push your body to the max' type programme.

And if you get the right balance, it can work brilliantly. If you get it slightly wrong, it can deplete your energy stores, increase carb and sugar cravings, and actually make your body HANG ON TO FAT even more! Ever started a new fitness routine and wondered why you weren't losing weight?

So what is the right type and amount of activity for hormone balance? Well that depends a lot on your own individual needs, health and circumstances. But I will explain how it affects your hormones and then you can jump to the MOVE section in Chapter 7 for the activities that help your hormones the most.

How does exercise affect your Feisty 4 hormones?

1. Exercise and cortisol

Lack of movement or too much sitting is a stress on the body. Circulation reduces, metabolism slows and fat storing increases. The right amount of regular exercise helps to reduce stress and improve mood. But too much exercise is also a stress on the body! Exercise raises cortisol and that's natural, but too much exercise when your energy reserves aren't enough can cause too much cortisol over time.

2. Exercise and insulin

Exercise has a direct effect on how insulin works. It increases your cells' response to insulin (something called sensitivity), and that's really important as it means that insulin can get into your cells to deliver the glucose it's carrying – and once in the cell it can be made into energy. When insulin can't get into the cell because the receptor isn't very sensitive to it, you can get insulin resistance, the precursor to diabetes. So exercise helps that whole process.

3. Exercise and thyroid

A sluggish circulation can impair the delivery of nutrients required for your thyroid to work properly (including iron). Lack of exercise slows your metabolism and can increase your fat:muscle ratio, further inhibiting your thyroid and fat-burning ability. Weight training or resistance work helps to build muscle, and muscle burns more energy than fat, so it helps your thyroid and your metabolism.

4. Exercise and oestrogen

Studies have shown that exercise helps to reduce your risk of breast cancer by reducing the amount of more dangerous oestrogen metabolites in the body. Extreme exercise however can increase cortisol and lower oestrogen too far, disrupting your regular cycle and weakening your bones.

Sitting around

Our modern lives make it difficult NOT to sit all day. According to a recent poll we spend an average of 56 hours a week sitting down – in our cars, at a desk, on the sofa. Many of us claim to have an active lifestyle. We might make it to the gym a few times a week. But unfortunately this doesn't seem to reduce the health risks of sitting for large portions of the day. Our bodies are not evolved to sit like this for as long as we do. And it's such a concern to the scientists that they have called it 'Sedentary Death Syndrome'!

We used to get exercise naturally from walking (we have cars now), housework (we have machines now) and hunting or growing food (we have supermarkets). Even keeping warm helped us burn extra calories (we now have central heating). So we have drifted into a habit of not moving. On top of that we sit at desks and computers for hours on end, hunched over and staring at a screen (I'm doing that right now!). For exercise we go to the gym or for a swim, and this kind of 'all or nothing' approach to activity can stress our system. Our bodies are designed to move regularly, with short bursts of energy and then rest.

What is so much sitting doing to you?

1. It slows down circulation, increasing your risk of heart disease and inhibiting nutrient, hormone and oxygen delivery to your cells
2. It increases risk of depression – less blood flow to the brain reduces key neurotransmitters like serotonin
3. It encourages fat storage – more insulin is released when your muscles are inactive, so more fat is locked up
4. It increases insulin resistance and risk of diabetes – more insulin floating around means your cells can become more resistant to it, eventually leading to diabetes
5. It accelerates ageing – exercise increases growth hormone, which helps to repair damage and keeps you young.

Over-exercising

Exercise raises cortisol, which is good if your body is not dealing with too much to start with! If you're already stressed or tired, that extra cortisol from over-exercising can end up depleting you, not recharging you. It can also increase the risk of muscle loss, frequent infections, risk of injury, fatigue and poor recovery. Your body can only take so much stress! If you're a gym bunny or addicted to long cardio, you need to review your routine, and take more rest if your hormones are out of whack.

And as for weight loss, for some people it seems the longer they exercise the more they DON'T lose weight! One study showed that those doing 30 minutes of exercise a day lost more weight than those doing an hour or more.

As a very basic rule, if exercise recharges your energy levels, it's an indication that it's doing you good. If you feel depleted afterwards, it may be taxing your adrenals and using up vital energy reserves. Best to do some gentle activity until your reserves are topped up.

Lack of sunlight

Feeling the warmth of the sun on your skin after a long winter is amazing isn't it? I think it's your body drinking in the vitamin D that it's been lacking for such a long time.

You know vitamin D is the 'sunshine vitamin' but did you know it is actually a hormone? And it's absolutely vital to keep you in optimal health.

According to the National Diet and Nutrition Survey, 90% of the general population in the UK have insufficient blood levels of vitamin D, and 5–20% of the population are in a state of severe deficiency.

Nearly every cell in your body has a vitamin D receptor, and more and more evidence is now confirming that its role in the body is much wider than just protecting your bones.

- **Immune booster** – vitamin D helps to fight infection. Maybe that's why we get more colds and flu in the wintertime when there's less sunlight
- **Autoimmune protection** – many conditions such as MS, Crohn's, rheumatoid arthritis, Hashimoto's and other autoimmune conditions have been linked to vitamin D deficiency
- **Cancer protection** – more and more evidence now points to the links between vitamin D deficiency and certain cancers, including breast, prostate and colon cancer. One study claims rates of these cancers would be cut by 50% if we got adequate amounts of vitamin D!
- **Bone and muscle health** – vitamin D regulates calcium levels and the activity of bone-building cells (severe deficiency we know causes rickets)
- **Brain health** – vitamin D activates the genes that release serotonin and dopamine, and deficiency can be a major

factor in mood disorders and depression. It also plays a crucial role in neurological health and cognitive function

- **Heart health** – vitamin D prevents calcium build-up in the arteries, helps to normalize blood pressure and reduce inflammation
- **Skin** – vitamin D helps to prevent excess cell proliferation (e.g. psoriasis, eczema)
- **Blood sugar balance and insulin control** – vitamin D helps to regulate blood sugar and prevent insulin resistance
- **Low sex drive** – vitamin D deficiency can cause low oestrogen and testosterone, which can affect your libido (may explain why you may feel more sexy in the summer?)

What can affect your vitamin D levels?

- **Lack of exposure to sunshine** – whether that is lack of actual sunshine all year round, covering up or avoiding the sun (or wearing sunblock)
- **Darker skin** – the darker your skin the more sun you need to be exposed to
- **Kidney or liver disease** – as vitamin D is converted in the liver and kidneys any issues here can lower your levels
- **Pregnancy** – you need extra amounts in pregnancy for building baby's bones
- **Stress** – cortisol is a steroid hormone made from cholesterol. If the body is stressed, cortisol will take priority over the synthesis of vitamin D
- **Obesity** – can reduce the biological activity of vitamin D
- **Genetics** – certain gene mutations can cause lower levels of vitamin D

If any of these affect you, then you will more than likely need to add a vitamin D3 supplement to your daily routine. Jump to Part 4 to find out more about supplements and testing.

SUMMARY

- Your diet can be a source of stress on your body
- Your hormones need the right nutrients to be produced, transported and metabolized
- Stress disrupts all your hormones
- Lack of sleep is directly affecting your energy, mood, weight and long-term health
- Are you exposed to endocrine-disrupting chemicals?
- Too little exercise AND too much exercise can disrupt your hormones
- If you're not getting enough sunlight, your hormones could be affected
- Smoking is not only highly toxic, it also messes with your hormones

CHAPTER 5

DITCH THE DIET – WHY DIETING AND EXTREME EXERCISE IS NOT WORKING FOR YOU ANY MORE

It's time to throw away the diet books that have been gathering dust on your bookshelves. Believe me it's going to feel amazing!

Trust me on this. I'm going to explain why dieting has to stop now you're over 40.

The Real Diet Story

I know how frustrating it is to be overweight and how you just want your fat to disappear fast. I have yo-yo dieted since I was a teenager. I know how it goes. You have a will of iron and go on a super low calorie diet – nowadays they come in easy meal replacement shakes – you don't even need to think about it. And they can work. You lose a few pounds and can fit into your jeans again. Then what happens? You go back to normal and the weight goes straight back on – AND MORE! And so you do it again. And each time you do one of these diets, your weight creeps up and up in the long term. This is so demoralizing, and you think it's your fault!

Low calorie and fad diets are designed for a quick fix – 'Lose 10lbs in three days' type thing. How many of us have fallen for them in the past? These diets can really stress your body and DISRUPT YOUR HORMONES!

I call this the Real Diet Story. The Before (wanting to lose say half a stone), the After (lost half a stone) and the After-After (put half a stone back on, PLUS another 5lbs). Now you're 12lbs heavier than when you stopped the diet.

> According to Zoe Harcombe, author of *The Obesity Epidemic*, 98% of people either don't lose weight on a calorie controlled diet, or regain what they lost. She also predicts that 90% of the UK population will be overweight or obese by 2050!

It's important to understand why diets do this. When you start a low calorie diet this restricts calories all of a sudden – so your brain thinks there is a famine happening, and after a while it alerts your adrenals to release cortisol to put your body into survival mode!

Cortisol starts to:

- break down your muscle (and some fat) to get sugar into your blood
- shut down your metabolism to conserve energy
- send constant signals to your brain that you need food desperately – anything to give you energy – so you get powerful carb and sugar cravings that you can't ignore

So you have no energy, your brain is foggy, you're losing muscle mass, you're CRAVING like mad and you're miserable!

You give in – you go back to your normal diet – but your metabolism is now really slow. So GUESS WHAT – you pile the weight back on – AND MORE.

These biochemical changes can last long after the diet has finished and could be the reason behind post-diet bingeing and the inevitable additional weight gain in the long term. It wasn't until I understood this that I realized what a great business model these mass slimming companies have. They are literally designed to keep you coming back over and over – clever huh?

If you want real sustainable results then you need to move away from the whole diet mentality and focus on your hormone balance instead.

Heena's story

Yo-yo diets

Heena was a 49-year-old business owner who had always been a yo-yo dieter, but couldn't shift her belly fat as she got older. Here's what she said after working with us:

'Once I hit 40, I found it really hard to lose weight. My usual diets just weren't working any more. I had no idea it could be down to my hormones! By ditching the foods that weren't serving my hormones, I managed to lose 10lbs of fat from my middle, I was able to stay awake past 9pm for the first time in years, and everyone noticed how glowing my skin was! And I finally have the energy and stamina to deal with stress. I'm amazed at what can be achieved in such a short time!'

Calories no more!

All calories are not equal

'Calories in, calories out…' is the message we've been told over and over for years. And of course calories matter, but they are not the whole story. In fact, for women over 40 they are even less relevant!

The calories in a handful of broccoli are not the same as the calories in a handful of popcorn. You know that already, because it just makes sense. But why isn't it factored into the message we're constantly given?

Because food is not just packages of calories. And your body is not like a bank account (in/out) – it's a chemistry lab!

Food is information, and it sends vital messages to your cells. Hormones don't respond to calories, they respond to nutrients.

Here's an example:

Take a large avocado at around 400 calories vs a Krispy Kreme doughnut at 200 calories.

On a calorie counting programme, officially you'd choose the doughnut!

But this is where the model is obviously flawed – it doesn't take into account what that food does to your biochemistry. Remember food is information right? So the nutrients in the avocado will tell the body to burn fat, whatever's in that doughnut will tell the body to store fat.

DIFFERENT MESSAGE – DIFFERENT OUTCOME!

If you are serious about controlling your hormones (and therefore your weight, energy, mood etc), you need to be thinking of food in a different way. Don't focus on the calorie content but rather the message this food has for your body. Then you are more likely to choose the foods that are going to nourish your hormones, increase your fat burning and boost your energy levels.

The big fat mistake

For YEARS, we've been told that FAT MAKES YOU FAT.

Ever since the 1950s when research came out that linked saturated fat and cholesterol with heart disease, the low-fat food industry has flourished and we have avoided dietary fat like the plague. It's so ingrained in us that most of us cringe at the thought of dripping or lard. Even BUTTER... ! And never touch the chicken skin, OMG!

The very sad thing is that the original research that started this all off has been invalidated. It turns out that saturated fat is not the main cause of heart disease. If that were the case, some high-fat eating populations around the world would have been wiped out. (One of these is the Inuit tribe of Greenland – they still eat high amounts of saturated animal fats, and have very low levels of heart disease, diabetes and obesity.)

The low-fat disaster

I've been on a ton of low-fat diets (like many women in their 40s!). They promise so much, and while I did lose weight initially, it always went back on (in spades!). And frankly they made me miserable! I now know why they are not a long-term solution...

- What do you replace the fat with? – The problem that the food industry had was that fat tastes good. So to take it out of a food meant putting something back that tasted good, and that was typically either sugar or artificial flavourings.
- Missing nutrients – real food contains many vital nutrients, including fat-soluble vitamins A, D, E and K. If you take the fat out of the food, you're not going to absorb these nutrients, putting you at risk of nutrient deficiencies.
- High carb – when you go low fat, you invariably choose carbs instead. Fat fills you up and carbs spike your blood sugar, causing the inevitable crash a couple of hours later, and another carb craving to replace the lost sugar. This leads to over-eating, excessive insulin and fat-storing.
- Low-fat diets have been shown to reduce HDL ('good' cholesterol) and increase triglycerides, risk factors for heart disease and diabetes.

Research has shown that snack foods with low-fat labels encouraged people to eat up to 50% more than those who saw labels without the low-fat claim.

And it's actually **low-carb** diets that have consistently performed better for weight loss in the general population. Balancing your blood sugar by limiting high-carb foods means that your metabolism works more efficiently and you are burning fat rather than storing it.

So should we all start eating higher fat diets again? Like our grandparents did?

For many of us, the answer is YES – simply put, FAT CAN BE YOUR FRIEND.

Why do we need fat?

- Cholesterol is the precursor of all your steroid hormones, and is vital for the production of bile and vitamin D
- Your brain is made up of 60% fat
- Every cell in your body needs fat for the membranes to work properly
- Fat is needed to dampen down inflammation and keep your immune system strong
- Fat helps to fill you up and prevent those between-meal sugar/carb cravings
- Fat helps you absorb your fat-soluble vitamins (A, D, E, K)

Without adequate fat, your hormones are going to suffer. And we know the critical role that hormones have in regulating metabolism, weight, energy, mood, brain function, fertility, libido, hunger, sleep and stress resilience. No wonder we can go a bit crazy on a low-fat diet!

But we all know that it's not quite that simple. All fat is not equal, and all people are not the same.

There are good and bad fats and obviously the bad ones we definitely need to avoid. And everyone has a different genetic make-up, meaning we all metabolize and absorb fat (and other nutrients) in different ways.

Types of fat

Fats are divided into three main groups:
- Saturated fatty acids (SAFAs) – short, medium and long chain
- Monounsaturated fatty acids (MUFAs) – medium and long chain
- Polyunsaturated fatty acids (PUFAs) – long chain

We have been told for years to avoid SAFAs and eat more MUFAs and PUFAs. Have a look at the list below. All foods that naturally contain fat have a mixture of different fats in them. You can't separate foods by different fat types. They all have a bit of everything. Which is why it is so ridiculous to say 'don't eat red meat – it's full of saturated fat'. It's also got PUFAs and MUFAs!

Food	Fat (g/100g)	% SaFAs	% MUFAs	% PUFAs
Beef	12	55	38	5
Rabbit	5.5	38	24	33
Cheddar Cheese	35	63	27	7
Butter	82	63	26	8
Salmon	11	18	40	28
Mackerel	16	21	50	21
Avocado	20	21	62	11
Sunflower Seeds	48	10	21	65
Almonds	56	8	68	19
Coconut Oil	100	87	6	1.5
Olive Oil	100	14	73	8

The 'good' fats

As you can see the above list are 'real foods'. Nature puts all the fats together in a food for a reason. We use them all for different things. Coconut oil for instance is the single biggest source of saturated fat, yet it is now recognized as a hugely beneficial food for our health.

The body can make most of the fats it needs, apart from Omega 3 and 6 fatty acids, which is why they are referred to as 'the essential fats'. This is why it's so vital to make sure you have enough in your diet and more importantly that they are both in balance. The problem is that the Omega 6 fats are plentiful in our modern diets (mainly from vegetable oils and animal products) and the Omega 3 fats are not as common (mainly from oily fish, some nuts and seeds). The ratio of Omega 6:3 fats has gone up in line with the increased intake of margarines and processed foods, and the relative decrease in oily fish consumption. Too high a ratio can increase inflammation in the body, and seriously mess with our hormones!

So it's important to make sure you are getting enough Omega 3s in your diet. Plant sources such as flaxseeds and walnuts aren't generally enough, as they need to go through a complex conversion process to get to the EPA and DHA Omega 3 fats that the body can use. If you're not eating oily fish (sardines, mackerel, salmon) regularly, you should consider a good quality supplement.

The 'bad' fats

When we start to mess with food by heating, processing, turning it into something convenient and increasing its shelf life, that's when the fat content can be problematic.

Processed foods and snacks are made with **vegetable oils**. Why? Because they are very cheap! But they are also very fragile, which means they can easily oxidize when heated or processed. To you and me, that means they go RANCID. And rancid oil promotes inflammation, cell damage and will do nothing for your waistline!

Here is a selection of foods containing 'bad fats':

- ready meals, sauces, salad dressings
- margarine or spread
- crisps and chips
- cookies, pastries, cakes, biscuits, snacks
- vegetable oils – e.g. soy, sunflower, canola, corn, grapeseed

Your unique biochemistry

Your genetic profile and health history is totally unique. Certain variations in your genes can alter the way you metabolize and absorb fats (and other nutrients). Equally, you can have problems digesting and absorbing fats due to other factors, such as nutrient deficiencies, underlying gut infections, inflammation, food sensitivities, stress and lifestyle factors.

So you may need to be careful with the total amount of fat in your diet. If you'd like to know more about genetic testing to identify your particular profile, contact us at www.happyhormonesforlife.com/contact.

So if you've been on low-fat diets before that haven't worked for you, go ahead and enjoy your organic crispy chicken skin, cook your sweet potatoes in goose fat, and eat lots of guilt-free avocados. Eating MORE fat might just help you LOSE fat.

- <u>Eat</u>: Grass-fed meat, free-range poultry, oily fish, organic full-fat dairy, eggs, nuts, seeds, avocados, olives, cold-pressed seed/nut oils.
- <u>Cook with</u>: Unrefined virgin coconut oil, lard, butter, goose/duck fat.
- <u>Avoid</u>: Processed foods, ready meals, fast foods, takeaways, margarine, 'low fat' foods, heated vegetable oils.

SUMMARY

- Low calorie and deprivation diets put your body into survival mode and can crush your metabolism
- Diets don't generally result in sustainable weight loss, you're more likely to put on even more afterwards
- Food is information not just calories

- You need to get away from the old calorie model and start focusing on foods that nourish your hormones
- The low-fat experiment is coming to an end (it has only resulted in more obesity!)
- Healthy fat is your friend (and it won't make you fat!)

CHAPTER 6

YOUR LIVER AND GUT – WHY THEY ARE IMPORTANT

> 'All disease begins in the gut. Bad digestion is the root of all evil.'
>
> Hippocrates 460 BC

Happy gut, happy hormones!

I'm not one to get excited about poo, but I'm a firm believer that health issues begin and end in the colon! In fact it's said that 90% of disease starts out as digestive issues.

You are not actually what you eat, you are what you **absorb**. You could be on the best diet in the world, but if your digestion isn't working optimally, you won't be absorbing those wonderful nutrients that make your hormones work properly!

And working with women's hormones week in week out, I see gut and digestive issues in 80% of my clients, even if they haven't come to see me for that.

That's because there's an inextricable link between hormone health and your gut function. Happy gut, happy hormones!

Do you have an unhealthy gut?

Here are some signs:

Constipation	Fungal infection	Bleeding gums
Flatulence	Bad breath	Indigestion
Food sensitivities	Heartburn	Foul-smelling stool
Nausea	Cramps	Blood/mucus in
Diarrhoea	Undigested food in	stool
Bloating	stool	Thrush

But very often you may not have any digestive issues at all. Microbial imbalances can cause symptoms anywhere in the body. Common ones include headaches, sinusitis, eczema, psoriasis, fatigue, brain fog, weight gain, mood swings, sugar cravings, joint pain and autoimmune conditions.

How does your gut health affect your Feisty 4 hormones?

1. Gut health and cortisol

We know that if your stress response is switched on, then digestive issues are more likely. It's not the body's priority to digest your food when a lion is attacking you (or more likely, you're sitting in a traffic jam)! Your digestive system is the home for your enteric nervous system (ENS), which is made up of more neurons than are found in the brain. It's capable of sensing, learning and remembering – and of course is where that 'gut feeling' comes from. Ever felt sick before an exam? That's the nerve cells in your gut reacting to stress. And that's why stress has such an impact on your digestive health (and digestive imbalances increase stress!). Information flows continuously back and forth between the brain and the gut via neurotransmitters – about 90% of which is going one way – gut to brain through your vagus nerve.

2. Gut health and insulin

If you've got too many bad bacteria or yeast in your gut, they can create cravings for sugar and carbs that can put you on the blood sugar roller coaster, stimulating lots of insulin release (and more fat storage!) and resulting blood sugar dips, which increase cortisol and impair digestion further.

3. Gut health and thyroid

Thyroid hormones need a variety of nutrients to function well, so if your digestive system isn't absorbing those nutrients your thyroid can suffer. Your T4 thyroid hormones also get converted into their T3 active form in your gut. And if you have leaky gut (see below), toxins and undigested foods can enter the bloodstream and attack your own tissue (this is one of the causes of autoimmune Hashimoto's thyroid disease).

4. Gut health and oestrogen

Your excess oestrogen needs to be eliminated through your liver and gut. There are a few things that can affect this clearance of oestrogen, causing it to be backed up and recirculated around the body. If you already have high circulating levels of oestrogen compared to progesterone, this can not only cause PMS and weight gain, but also put you at higher risk of oestrogen-driven conditions such as fibroids, endometriosis and breast and ovarian cancer. Factors that affect the clearance of oestrogen include dysbiosis (gut flora imbalances), constipation, stress, environmental toxins, alcohol and a low fibre/high sugar diet.

Did you know?

Your intestines are about 22 feet long (nearly 7 metres) – the surface area would cover almost 3000 square feet, the size of a tennis court!

There's a good reason for its size – your digestive system is vital for your survival. It's your nutrient feed, your main defence system, your main elimination route for waste, and the location for a million different vital biochemical processes.

Over 70% of your immune system is located in your digestive tract. It makes sense for it to be there if you think about it. It's your main barrier against letting anything 'foreign' from entering your internal system. And it does an amazing job, day in day out, dealing with chemicals, bacteria, viruses, that you don't want in your system.

How does it work?

When you eat something, your digestive process starts in your mouth with saliva and chewing, and finishes in your colon when you eliminate it. Along the way, it will absorb what your body needs and keep out the rest. To do this well, you need everything to be working. You need to produce enough digestive enzymes and stomach acid so that your food can be broken down properly. You need your digestive tract to be contracting well so that your food can move down efficiently. You need to have a nicely integral gut wall that can absorb all the nutrients but keep out the 'foreign' stuff. You need your gut bacteria to be nicely balanced so that it keeps your immune system working well and your hunger hormones in check.

So it's a very complex process, and therefore things can go wrong along the way.

What can go wrong?

1. Gut flora imbalance (or dysbiosis)
You are made up of trillions of bacteria and microbes (latest guess is 100 trillion)! In fact it is thought that microbial cells

outnumber human cells by 3 to 1 in our bodies! So you are essentially just a host for the critters. And they play a vital role in your health:

- keeping the 'bad' microbes in check
- regulating digestive function, keeping everything working well
- acting as immune protection
- keeping the gut barrier intact and working properly
- producing vital nutrients
- regulating your hormones

Your gut flora is made up of millions of different strains of microbes – good and bad. This environment (called your microbiome) is totally unique to you and extremely delicately balanced. The good and bad live together harmoniously, all with jobs to do.

Unfortunately, many of us have (unknowingly) altered our microbiomes with antibiotics, poor dietary choices, medications and stress.

You see when the balance is altered the bad guys can overgrow and take over. This is generally not good news and we suffer the consequences with digestive issues, increased infection and the problems that brings.

2. Low stomach acid

Without enough stomach acid you can't digest your food properly. Hydrochloric acid and digestive enzymes are secreted when you start to eat (actually even before you eat, with smell and anticipation). The acid and enzymes start to break down the food (especially protein) before it passes into the small intestine. If proteins are not digested properly, they can sit in the gut too long, causing gas, bloating and indigestion. The body can also react to these foreign particles and cause an immune reaction.

Low acid can also impair carbohydrate breakdown, causing undigested carbs to ferment in the stomach and small intestines – and this feeds bad bacteria, causing them to overgrow. This can result in more lasting digestive issues.

Factors involved in low stomach acid include age, stress, infection (e.g. H. pylori), indigestion drugs (PPIs, antacids) and nutrient deficiencies (e.g. zinc).

3. Food intolerances

Certain foods can cause your own body to react against them and launch an immune response. Food can be seen as dangerous if for example you don't have the enzyme required to digest it (e.g. lactose), or it has a component that can aggravate the immune system (e.g. gluten). When the immune system is activated, it uses inflammation just like it would if you had injured yourself. Except you can't see it, it's on the inside of your gut! It does all sorts of damage though – it stops you absorbing all your nutrients, and it can make holes in your gut lining so that toxins and food particles can go through unchecked. Inflammation can spread to all parts of the body and can cause more serious chronic conditions.

4. Leaky gut

Food intolerances, gut flora imbalances and stress can cause the gut lining to become 'leaky'. This is called intestinal permeability, and it can result in undigested food particles, chemicals and bacterial waste leaking through your digestive tract and entering your bloodstream. These foreign particles stimulate your immune system to react, promoting inflammation and raising cortisol. This is now thought to be at the root of many autoimmune conditions such as rheumatoid arthritis, lupus (SLE), diabetes type 1, Hashimoto's thyroiditis, coeliac disease, Crohn's disease and many more.

Depression and sleep

Did you know that most of your serotonin (happy hormone) is produced in your gut, not your brain? That's because it's needed to help with gut motility (keeping you moving). But we also know how vital serotonin is for your mood and sleep – and it's also the precursor to melatonin, your sleep hormone. So if your gut isn't working as well as it should, it can affect your production of serotonin and increase your risk of mood disorders, depression and poor sleep.

Are antidepressants the answer?

Most antidepressants are SSRIs – selective serotonin reuptake inhibitors – that means they keep the serotonin you produce from naturally degrading so you have more of it for longer. Which is great, for a while, but they're not meant to be taken long term. So wouldn't it make more sense to investigate gut health to see why serotonin production might be lower than it should be? It does to me!

The impact of modern life

Diet

Refined carbs and sugar – too much can help to feed the bad guys in the gut, crowding out the beneficial microbes.

Low fibre – 'good' bacteria prefer fibre to sugar, so the more fibre you eat, the more you are helping your good bacteria. Fibre not only helps you feel full and slows down sugar absorption, but it also helps to eliminate that excess oestrogen.

Low probiotic foods – for centuries, many cultures have used fermentation as a way of preserving foods. This gave them a constant source of good bacteria and probiotics in their diets. These days we have to go out of our way to find fermented foods, either making it ourselves (it's actually really easy) or buying it ready made. And this dietary change has had a big impact on our gut flora balance.

Food processing – the food additives, preservatives and colourings that are routinely used in processed foods can cause inflammation in your digestive system, which in turn can alter the delicate balance between absorbing nutrients and keeping out toxins.

Gluten and other common 'aggravators' – sometimes your immune system inappropriately reacts to things it is exposed to. This can result in outright allergies (such as peanut, pollen, dust mites, coeliac disease, etc) or it can cause a less acute reaction, often labelled an 'intolerance' or 'sensitivity', which can cause digestive issues but also more systemic issues such as headaches, joint pain, fatigue, skin issues and hormone imbalances. Gluten, dairy, soy, corn and eggs are the top five common food intolerances, but of course you can be sensitive to any food.

Gluten and hormones – I have noticed in clinic that women with gluten sensitivity seem to suffer more during perimenopause. As sex hormones start to decline, resulting imbalances can be made worse by eating gluten. Inflammation in the gut caused by gluten tends to feed inflammation (pain) in the surrounding areas (your reproductive system!), as well as raising cortisol, which further decreases sex hormone production and puts a strain on the thyroid. Inflammation in the gut can also affect your serotonin levels, affecting your mood and your sleep.

Alcohol – not only gives you more of a hangover as you get older, but it can also irritate your gut lining and impair your liver function, increasing circulating oestrogen.

Mindless eating

A survey done by Conscious Food found that we average six, eight and nine minutes to eat breakfast, lunch and dinner respectively! A measly 23 minutes eating food in a day. How often do you grab food while you work, watch TV or chat on the phone? Do you even know you're eating? I have often eaten something without even realizing I'm doing it (popcorn and Pringles are particularly good at that!).

This kind of eating puts a huge stress on your digestive system and can increase your cortisol levels. It makes you skip an important stage of your digestive process, the cephalic stage. This is when the brain anticipates food and signals the body to get ready by producing saliva and digestive enzymes. Without this preparation, it's harder to properly digest your food. On top of that, your 'feel full' signals take more time to get to the brain, so you are likely to eat more.

But research has shown that slowing everything down can help to support your digestion, reduce cortisol levels and increase weight loss.

Eating on the run, bolting food down and not chewing properly can all cause:

- increased or decreased gut motility (i.e. you can get diarrhoea and/or constipation), which impairs absorption of those hormone-friendly nutrients
- decreased stomach acid, which can hinder protein digestion

- an imbalance of good and bad bacteria, leaving you more vulnerable to infection
- inflammation in the gut wall, making it more prone to leaks (and letting in toxins)

Medications

Overuse of antibiotics – I think this is changing (probably due to the fact that the bugs are mostly now resistant), but doctors are still over-prescribing broad spectrum antibiotics – the ones that wipe out ALL your bacteria, good and bad. If you have a bacterial infection then of course you need them to get rid of it. But I've seen people taking them for a sore throat most likely caused by a virus (they don't work on viruses!). These are not harmless drugs. They kill all your bacteria. We need bacteria (we are 90% made up of them!). The good bacteria help us survive; they are part of our immune system. I'm not against antibiotics for the right reasons, but make sure you know why you are taking them and take a good quality probiotic two hours after your antibiotic dose.

Every time you swallow a broad spectrum antibiotic, you are killing off not just the bad guys causing the infection (if there is one) but also the good beneficial bacteria that you need. That leaves the coast clear for yeast to take control (and in my clinic I'm seeing a huge rise in the number of candida infections).

Other medications like anti-inflammatory painkillers and synthetic hormones can damage the gut lining, impair absorption of nutrients and risk leakage of waste and toxins into the bloodstream.

Janine's story

Gluten sensitive

Janine is a 47-year-old English teacher who was really fed up. She had tried every fad diet and sweating at the gym four times a week – none of it touched the layers of fat around her middle. She was exhausted every afternoon and struggled to get on with day-to-day tasks. When we took gluten out of her diet, things changed dramatically for her. Here's what she said after her programme:

'I have learnt so much: the impact of years of low-fat restricted dieting and, unexpectedly, the negative impact of gluten in my diet. Eliminating it and reintroducing it was revelatory. Brain fog! I didn't even know that was a 'thing'. Before taking gluten out of my diet I couldn't even remember the pin number of the bank card I had been using for 25 years! And finally, I have lost much of the fat around my middle.... I even tucked a top in my jeans the other day! Every day I look forward to looking after myself because I know now how to do it!'

Your liver

When you hear the word detoxification, it usually brings up images of exotic juice fasts or powders that leave you sitting on the loo all day.

But your body has its own detoxification system – your liver. And everything you eat and drink gets into your bloodstream and eventually passes through the liver.

It's an amazing thing your liver – did you know it's the largest organ in the body, weighing over four pounds? And if you lost three-quarters of it, it would regenerate into a whole new liver?

And it has so many jobs to do. Over 500 at the last count.

Are you looking after it? That doesn't just mean watching how many glasses of wine you're drinking.

Of course that's important, but did you know that as well as detoxing the alcohol, your liver also regulates your hormones? And deals with all the chemicals you are exposed to (that includes the perfume you spray on, the chlorine in your tap water, the pills you take and the pesticides on your fruit and veg?).

Your liver is working harder than ever. Over the last few decades, it has had to deal with thousands of new chemicals in the air you breathe, the food you eat, the products you use and the water you drink. And clear up that nightly glass or two of wine!

Your genes play a huge part in how well you detoxify and some people can tolerate a huge number of toxins with no apparent effects. However, for many women, these chemicals can cause huge disruption, especially and worryingly to your hormones.

And when your liver struggles to cope, toxins and waste can get backed up (like a Hoover bag full of dust) and they can get recirculated back into our bloodstream.

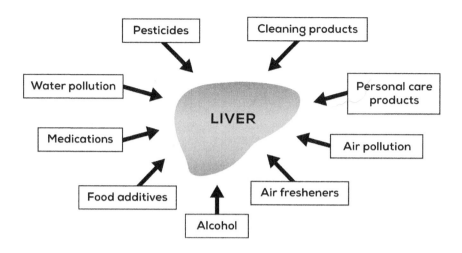

How does that affect your hormones?

1. **Too much oestrogen?** One important role of the liver is to get rid of excess oestrogen, a very important process as too much oestrogen can cause PMS, heavy periods, breast tenderness, bloating, weight gain and headaches. You might also have a build-up of more dangerous metabolites of oestrogen, the ones that can cause breast cancer and other chronic diseases.

2. **Low thyroid?** Your liver is where a lot of your thyroid hormones get converted into active mode, so if the liver is struggling, a deficiency of active thyroid hormones can slow down your metabolism, hang on to fat stores and crash your energy levels. And equally a sluggish thyroid inhibits liver function! And round you go again…

3. **Blood sugar roller coaster?** Your liver plays a vital role in blood sugar balance. If your diet is too carb heavy, or you have a lot of stress going on, your liver can struggle to regulate your blood sugar which can cause fatigue, sugar cravings, fat storage (especially belly fat), mood swings and brain fog.

On top of that, your liver:

- provides nutrients – converting fats, carbs and proteins into nutrients the body can use
- stores nutrients – such as fat-soluble vitamins and minerals
- stores sugar – for quick release when we are stressed
- makes toxins safe so that you can eliminate them and they don't mess with your hormones
- makes cholesterol so you can make steroid hormones

This is a fraction of what the liver has to do, so you need to make sure you're looking after it.

Find out more about how to love your liver in Step 3 of the Happy Hormone Code in Chapter 7.

---

10 tips to love your liver

1. Drink more water, less alcohol! Now you don't need me to tell you this one, it's a no-brainer, but as you get older your liver is less able to cope with alcohol, and hydration is even more important (just saying…!)
2. Eat more broccoli – and cauliflower, kale, cabbage, Brussels sprouts, rocket, watercress – they are all cruciferous veg that are loaded with something called indole-3-carbinol which helps to detoxify that excess oestrogen. Aim for two portions a day (if you can't manage that, DIM is the supplement that does a similar thing).
3. Ditch the sugar, refined carbs and processed foods – stressing out your liver with too much sugar and industrial fats is going to raise insulin, cortisol and oestrogen – not good news!

4. Eat enough protein – a protein shake is an easy way to do this. Make sure it's a good quality protein (plant based if you are dairy intolerant).

5. Get your bowels moving – if you're constipated, your toxic waste is going to build up, and guess what? Your oestrogen is going to get recycled. So eat plenty of fibre, supplement with magnesium, drink plenty of water and exercise daily.

6. Watch the pill popping – don't just pop a pill without thought! Your liver has to detox any kind of medication, including paracetamol, ibuprofen, birth control pills and indigestion tablets.

7. Reduce stress – make time for your food (try mindful eating), balance your cortisol by practising daily relaxation techniques (mindfulness, deep breathing, long baths, music).

8. Switch your personal and household products to natural organic ones – what you put on your skin goes straight into your bloodstream. Put your product into the App 'Think Dirty' to see how 'toxic' it is.

9. Go organic – reduce your exposure to harmful pesticides and other mass chemicals by switching to organic for fruit, veg, dairy, eggs and meat where possible.

10. Get a sweat on! Sweating is a great way to get rid of toxins. The skin is one of your most important detoxification organs. Exercise, saunas, steam rooms – try anything that gets your sweat dripping.

SUMMARY

- Your gut is vital for all aspects of your health
- Only 10% of your DNA is human, the rest is microbial!
- Your gut microbes have a big impact on your appetite, weight, sleep, metabolism, immune system, mood, focus, memory and much more
- Stress and eating on the run can ruin your digestion and cause inflammation and leaky gut
- Your liver is working harder than ever to keep you clean and healthy (it has over 500 different functions)
- If your liver and gut are under strain, your hormones will be affected

PART 3

YOUR HORMONE-BALANCING PLAN

CHAPTER 7

THE HAPPY HORMONE CODE – YOUR SIMPLE FOUR-STEP NUTRITION AND LIFESTYLE SOLUTION

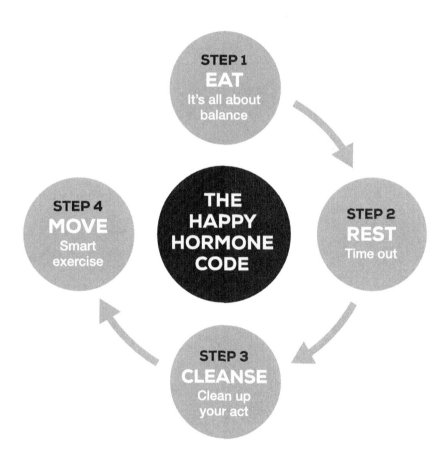

So you've learnt about your main Feisty 4 hormones and the dietary and lifestyle factors that can affect them. Now it's time to learn how to regain control of them, so that you can enjoy the benefits for years to come.

My four-step Happy Hormone Code is a simple nutrition and lifestyle solution designed to get your hormones working for you, not against you. It's a system you can use as your foundation for happy hormones for life.

Because when your 'Feisty 4' are nicely balanced, you will feel great. You will be at your ideal weight, full of energy, with balanced moods, a clear head and be able to handle stress with ease.

My system is a culmination of many years of study and practice into the latest cutting-edge research, tools and techniques into what works for hormone health.

Hormones need nutrient-dense foods, rest and repair time, a clean environment and a healthy active body. If you follow these steps you can give your hormones the tools they need to look after you back.

> *'It's easier to rebalance your hormones than live with the misery of hormone imbalances.'*
> Dr Sara Gottfried, author of The Hormone Cure

Multiply the benefits
This system has health benefits for everyone – you don't have to have a hormone imbalance to live this way. These principles will help everyone to live a more healthy life. If you can get your partners, kids, friends and families eating this way, they are only going to benefit too!

STEP 1 – EAT

Food is Step 1 for a reason. It's the one thing that you can do right away and you can feel the difference really quickly. That's because food directly affects our biochemistry and our hormone balance – almost immediately.

To truly balance your hormones, you need to start seeing food differently. Not as calories, but as INFORMATION. Food has the power to change how you look, feel, think and perform. It does this by sending messenger signals to your cells and hormones. It can literally tell your body to burn or store fat, to increase or decrease your energy levels, to alter your mood, to change how your brain functions or to switch on genes that cause disease.

So on my programmes we focus on the foods that nourish your hormones – and we don't count calories!

Because if you give your hormones all the nutrients they need, they can work properly and be in balance. When that happens, your body can relax – nutrients are plentiful, so no need to stress out. And a relaxed body can release excess weight and restore your metabolism – giving you more energy, balancing out your moods and providing energy to your brain, skin, heart and all your organs.

All without having to deprive or exhaust yourself. And you certainly won't go hungry!

I know it can be difficult to get away from convenience eating. When I started down this path I had no time to think about eating real food. I'm a mum of two children, I run my own business, and at the same time try to plan healthy meals, exercise regularly – not to mention maintaining some semblance of a social life! I thought it was so much easier to put a ready meal in the microwave…

It wasn't until I actually started to feed my hormones the right nutrients that I realized it actually made life a lot simpler – AND made me feel a whole lot better. And it wasn't just about me either; this benefited the whole family.

Everything changed for me once I started to eat real food. The tyre around my middle disappeared; I could fit into my old clothes again (the ones I had been keeping 'just in case'). I suddenly had enough energy to get through the day and stay awake at night to watch a film with my husband (all the way to the end!). I was so much calmer and nicer to the kids and everyone around me. And my brain fog disappeared almost overnight – all from eating the right foods, and tweaking my lifestyle.

And I'd really love that to happen to every woman over 40 who is struggling with similar issues.

So let's have a closer look at what hormones need for optimal production, storage, transport and excretion.

Hormone-friendly foods

These are the main food groups that form the basis of my programmes. These foods will give you the macronutrients and micronutrients that your hormones need, as well as some essential phytonutrients that will boost their performance.

While I don't want you to worry or stress over portion sizes, you should listen to your body. It takes time for the satiety hormones in your stomach to send the message to your brain that you've had enough, so eat slowly and stop when you're around 80% full. If your appetite hormones are a bit out (which can happen when you're overweight or stressed), then use the Happy Hormones Plate as a guide for proportions.

Low GL (Glycaemic Load) foods – e.g. fruit, veg, wholegrains, beans, pulses, meat, fish, eggs, nuts, seeds – these foods release sugar more slowly into the blood, thereby keeping blood sugar levels more stable. This helps to avoid excess insulin in your system, which can disrupt your other hormones and cause symptoms such as cravings, PMS, fatigue, brain fog and mood swings. It also helps to reduce your fat stores (insulin is your fat-storing hormone!). See Resources for a Low GL guide.

Vegetables – as many varieties and colours as possible! They will supply plenty of vitamins, minerals, phytonutrients and fibre. Aim to fill half your plate with colourful veg at each meal, and rotate often.

Get to know your cruciferous veg!

A family of vegetables known as cruciferous vegetables are super helpful for your hormones, especially your oestrogen. They contain indole-3-carbinol, a substance that helps metabolize and eliminate excess oestrogen, which can contribute towards PMS, headaches, bloating, breast tenderness, painful periods and an increased risk of PCOS, fibroids, endometriosis and breast/ovarian cancer. They include broccoli, cauliflower, cabbage, collard greens, kale, bok (or pak) choy, rocket, watercress, radish, Brussels sprouts, mustard seeds, wasabi, horseradish.

Fibre – e.g. wholegrains, veg, fruit, oats, beans, seeds. Fibre protects you from the blood sugar roller coaster (and therefore reduces insulin and fat storing!) by slowing down the release of sugar from the carbs in your meal. It also helps you get rid of waste, toxins and excess oestrogen. Aim for a minimum of 35g a day. That might look like this:

- 1 apple (5g)
- 1 cup lentils (15g)
- 2 tbsp flaxseeds (5g) or 1 tbsp chia seeds (5g)
- 1 cup broccoli (5g)
- ½ avocado (5g)

You can always add some soluble fibre to your daily smoothie in the form of psyllium husk.

Good fats – e.g. nuts, seeds, olives, avocado, oily fish, organic dairy, eggs, organic meat, olive oil, coconut oil. These fats are essential for the production, storage and transport of your hormones. Cholesterol is the precursor to all steroid hormones (that's why low cholesterol can be very damaging). You also need fat in your food to absorb the vitamins that are fat soluble (A, D, E and K). It's no good drinking skimmed milk, as you won't absorb any of these vitamins! Please avoid all low-fat foods from now on – if they take the fat out, they often replace it with sugar or artificial flavourings, which will do you more harm. So embrace healthy fats – enjoy your chicken skin, cream, butter, eggs and streaky bacon (organic of course!) – and remember this most of all: good fat doesn't make you fat!

Why I love coconut oil

The stuff that looks like lard and is full of saturated fats, right? Yes, it is made up of saturated fat. HOWEVER it's the type of fat that is important.

Two thirds of its fats are medium chain triglycerides (MCTs), as opposed to the long chain triglycerides (LCTs) that are abundant in most other fats we consume. MCTs are treated very differently in the body and are thought to have many health benefits. Current research into the potential role of coconut oil in weight loss is particularly exciting.

The oil is derived from the white meat of the coconut, which is cold pressed into oil and has been used in South East Asia and the Pacific for centuries for eating, medicine and skin treatments. The coconut is so valued by the people of the Pacific Islands that they call it 'the tree of life'.

Coconut oil can be helpful in boosting your metabolism and stabilizing blood sugar.

Potential health benefits

- Instant energy – MCTs are smaller than LCTs so do not need to pass through bile salts in the gut to be digested, they go straight to the liver to be quickly metabolized into ketone bodies to provide instant energy. They are not stored like other fats and are the preferred energy source for cells. This can result in a surge of energy and an increase in metabolism (a benefit for underactive thyroids and weight loss).
- Weight loss – as well as boosting metabolism, MCTs have been shown to increase satiety after eating so you feel full for longer, reducing your cravings for sugary snacks. Many studies are showing promising results for reducing obesity.
- Antimicrobial and antifungal – almost half the fat content is made up of lauric acid, which converts in the body to monolaurin, a substance that can attack viruses, bacteria and fungi. There are very few dietary sources of lauric acid (the main one being breast milk!). It can be effective against candida and other microbial overgrowths.

- Anti-ageing and heart health – coconuts contain polyphenol antioxidants that have been shown to protect the liver against free radicals, support the immune system and protect against cardiovascular disease. One antioxidant called p-Coumaric acid is associated with arterial protection and decreasing LDL cholesterol. These compounds also contain vitamin E, a known heart protector and scavenger of free radicals.
- Brain health – in Alzheimer's disease, brain cells are starved of glucose due to insulin resistance. Ketone bodies provided by MCTs can be an alternative source of fuel, with the potential to reduce symptoms and worsening of the disease.
- Diabetes – MCTs act like glucose as an instant source of energy, but they don't cause an insulin spike, the major contributing factor over time for insulin resistance and diabetes. Increasing metabolic rate also improves insulin levels. Eating fat with carbs helps slow the release of sugar into the blood. This helps reduce insulin and balance blood sugar, lowering the risk of developing insulin resistance and diabetes.

Tips for using coconut oil

- In smoothies – not only does it taste great, but also the fat will help you absorb all the other great nutrients in the smoothie (as long as there are lots of green veggies in there!).
- In coffee! I love a teaspoon in my morning coffee. It gives me a double dose of energy and focus first thing. Amazingly delicious too, blended up with a little almond milk.
- In cooking – many vegetable, plant and seed oils are unstable and can denature when exposed to high

temperatures (frying, roasting), turning the oil into trans-fats. Coconut oil is perfect for cooking as it is very stable and does not change structure, even at very high temperatures.

- And remember, all coconut oil is not equal! It's important to buy the cold-pressed organic extra virgin variety as it is not heated during the extraction process, so retains its antioxidants and avoids rancidity.

Protein – e.g. organic meat, fish, dairy, eggs, nuts, seeds, beans, lentils, quinoa, soy, spirulina, protein shakes. Good quality protein can help slow the release of sugar into the blood (reducing excess insulin), boost your metabolism, increase satiety hormones (making you eat less) and repair bone and muscle. It is also essential for your detoxification process. That's why I recommend protein at each meal, especially breakfast. Good sources are eggs, nut-based muesli or granola (low sugar), organic natural yoghurt and protein green smoothies.

Organic – where possible, choose organic produce. So much evidence now proves that pesticides used in conventional farming can mess with your hormones. For fruit and veg especially choose organic where you eat the skin, such as apples, berries, plums, etc. Don't worry too much about bananas, avocados or pineapples, as you will avoid most of the chemicals when you peel them. Non-organic animal produce may contain fewer nutrients and stimulate inflammatory pathways in the body. Choose grass-fed and organic meat, fish, dairy and eggs. I realize it's not always possible, but if you try to get the best food you can afford it will pay dividends.

Dark chocolate! – the cocoa bean is full of antioxidants and many hormone-friendly minerals like magnesium. Watch the sugar content though, the darker the better (over 70% is preferable).

Protein smoothies – my belief and experience is that if you get to start your day with a nutritious smoothie that happens to taste great as well, not only are you getting a great hit of nutrients early on, but you will also be more likely to eat more healthily for the rest of the day. Good smoothies are very filling too which should help prevent the mid-morning cravings you can get after a carb-heavy breakfast. Always favour green ingredients over fruit (to avoid a blood sugar hit) and make sure you add protein and a healthy fat to give you the full range of macronutrients. The fat will also help you absorb all those lovely vitamins and minerals.

You can follow this general guide to make your own or check out my favourite smoothie recipes in the Recipes section.

Liquid base: filtered water, coconut water or milk base (organic full-fat milk, unsweetened almond milk, organic soy milk, oat milk, coconut milk, nut milk)

Fruit (maximum two of these): ½ banana, handful of berries, ½ apple, ½ pear, kiwi, ¼ pineapple, ¼ mango

Veg (as much as possible): e.g. kale, chard, lettuce, rocket, salad leaves, cabbage, fennel, ginger, cucumber, celery

Herbs and spices: e.g. mint, parsley, coriander, cinnamon, vanilla, turmeric

Protein: either whey-based protein powder (make sure it's organic and made from grass-fed cows) or dairy-free, plant-based protein powder (I like pea protein but there are lots of others)

Fats: any nuts (unprocessed and raw), seeds (flax, chia, sunflower, pumpkin, sesame, hemp), avocado, coconut oil, flax oil, hempseed oil, olive oil

<u>Optional add-ins:</u> see smoothie recipes for all sorts of superfood options.

Coffee and tea – I know how much some of you love your coffee (me included!), and in the past I have left it out of my programmes. BUT recent research is overwhelmingly clear that good quality real coffee has some significant health benefits, and can even prevent diabetes and other chronic diseases. So I do not universally discourage coffee and tea drinking. HOWEVER, there are some caveats here:

- it has to be real coffee not instant (we are staying away from processed foods, remember?)
- if you want to switch to decaf, make sure it's not made using chemicals (go for the Swiss Water or CO_2 method of extraction)
- if coffee makes you jittery, anxious, gives you palpitations or you have trouble sleeping, it's best to avoid it. Some of us are genetically not great detoxifiers of caffeine and have to limit our consumption.
- if you have a dairy intolerance, you need to drink it without milk. I love my real coffee with frothed up coconut milk – it's delicious.

Hydration – water is very underrated! The average female is 55% water. Every cell needs water, and hormones need it to be transported around the body. Water helps digestion and detoxification and increased water intake has also been shown to help with weight loss. And most of us are dehydrated (which is a major stress on the body – hello cortisol!).

Every person needs different amounts, but a good target is to try to drink 2 litres (3.5 pints) of water a day (including herbal teas) and you know you're hydrated when your urine is pale. It helps if you drink a pint of water when you wake up – add some lemon juice to it to kickstart your liver! Then keep a bottle or jug topped up throughout the day that you can sip (avoiding plastic if possible). Adding cucumber, lemon or mint to the water gives it a refreshing taste. Make sure it's filtered water (or bottled), as tap water can contain hormone-disrupting chemicals, such as fluoride, chlorine and heavy metals.

Phytoestrogens – these are plant nutrients that research has shown help with oestrogen balance. They are very similar to our own oestrogen molecules so can act as oestrogen regulators. The main ones in our diet are the isoflavones from the soy bean, along with flaxseeds, beans, lentils, chickpeas. Flaxseeds are the best source of lignans, which help to bind waste oestrogen (100 x more than any other food!), followed by sesame seeds, cruciferous veg, wholegrains and fruit.

Superfoods

1. **Acai berry** – pronounced (ah-sigh-ee) is a traditional part of the Amazonian diet. Rich in fibre, essential fats and one of the highest scoring superfoods for antioxidants.
2. **Baobab** – native to Africa, this fruit is packed with vitamin C, six times more than an orange! But it also has six times more potassium than a banana, and twice as much calcium as milk.
3. **Chlorella and spirulina** – both blue-green algae, they have a super high nutrient content, and are natural detoxifiers. Not the best tasting foods I'm afraid, so best taken in capsule form or added to a green smoothie.
4. **Hibiscus** – not strictly a superfood, more of a super tea! I recently learnt that the hibiscus flower has over three times more antioxidant strength than green tea! So I now brew up a large jug of hibiscus tea (you can get lots of different flavours), let it cool, add some stevia, and keep it in the fridge to sip on during the day. It's a bit like fruit squash!

---

5. **Goji berries** – also called wolfberries – have long been used in Chinese medicine for all kinds of health issues, including anti-ageing. Apart from tasting good (think chewy little red raisins but not so sweet), they are packed full of antioxidants, vitamins, minerals and protein.

6. **Lucuma** – from the lucuma fruit in South America, rich in fibre, vitamins and minerals, it is really useful to use as a natural sweetener due to its caramel flavour.

7. **Maca powder** – a Peruvian root, maca has been used for centuries for energy, stamina and sex drive – it's known as 'nature's Viagra' in Peru!

8. **Matcha** – a concentrated powdered green tea, matcha has three times the antioxidants of standard green tea. Great to add to creamy porridge, smoothies or as an alternative to your usual coffee latte.

9. **Moringa** – known as Africa's Miracle Tree, the moringa leaf is packed with vital hormone-balancing nutrients and is a great source of plant protein. It's also rich in fibre, which helps with detoxification and elimination of excess oestrogen. And the high levels of magnesium help to improve mood and relieve stress.

10. **Raw cacao** – chocolate in its raw form is not only the most delicious food on earth (in my humble opinion!) but is also one of the most healthy too (there is a chocolate god!). High levels of antioxidants and magnesium are its main strengths, but the ability to make everything taste good in a smoothie has to be up there too.

11. **Wheatgrass** – wheatgrass is rich in chlorophyll, the green pigment from plants that helps with detoxification and is a known DNA protector. Another acquired taste (read disgusting), but disguise it in a smoothie or neck it down in a shot like tequila!

Healthy swaps

Swap white rice for brown, wild rice or cauliflower rice
Swap couscous for quinoa
Swap spaghetti for courgetti (spiralized courgettes)
Swap white potatoes for sweet potatoes
Swap pasta for gluten-free brown rice pasta
Swap fruit yoghurts for organic natural yoghurt (full-fat)
Swap fizzy drinks, fruit juice or squash for sparkling water
with fresh lemon
Swap noodles for rice or buckwheat noodles
Swap soy sauce (contains gluten) for tamari
Swap peanut butter for almond or cashew butter
Swap fruit smoothies for green smoothies
Swap white sugar for coconut sugar or maple syrup
Swap biscuits for oatcakes
Swap cereal for eggs or oats
Swap white wine for red
Swap salad dressings for home-made olive oil/lemon juice
or vinegar
Swap wheat flour for gluten-free flours (almond, coconut,
rice, tapioca, millet, buckwheat, amaranth, arrowroot, chia,
chickpea or gram, quinoa, teff)

So you know what hormones love, now you need to know what
they don't thrive on! Here are the main things to avoid.

Hormone-disrupting foods

These are some of the foods that you need to be limiting as they
don't serve your hormones well and can increase stress in your
body.

Sugar! – of course you want to avoid sugar, as it upsets your blood sugar balance and causes excessive insulin release. It's not just the obvious white stuff that you need to avoid though; watch out for hidden sugars in processed foods, ready meals, baked goods, fruit smoothies, juices and LOW FAT products. Start reading labels. And don't swap for DIET products – these contain artificial sweeteners that can affect hormones (especially in the gut and brain).

Sugar and sugar alternatives

There are lots of different types of sugar out there jumping on the anti-sugar bandwagon and claiming to be a healthier alternative. At the end of the day, sugar is sugar! But there are some sugars that are preferable to refined sugars, and there are some that you need to avoid. Here's my list:

AVOID
- White and brown sugar – refined, processed.
- Fructose – initially thought to be healthier due to its low GI index, but fructose goes straight to the liver and deposits as fat.
- Honey – processed honey may seem a better option, but all the goodness has gone and what you've got left is pure sugar.
- Agave syrup – don't be fooled by the 'healthy' label often attributed to agave. It's pure fructose and highly processed.
- Xylitol (also erythritol and sorbitol) – these are sugar alcohols which are not digested by the body, and don't generally raise blood sugar levels. However, they are highly processed and can cause digestive issues, so are best avoided. (Highly toxic to dogs by the way!)

- Evaporated cane juice – often included in packaged foods, this is just sugar cane syrup in disguise.

PREFERABLE (in moderation)
- Raw honey – in its raw form, honey retains lots of nutrients and antioxidants.
- Organic maple syrup – a good alternative to other sugar products, as it doesn't go through much processing and it has a good nutrient profile. The darker versions are more nutrient dense.
- Coconut sugar (or palm sugar) – also in the form of coconut syrup or nectar, it's rich in nutrients (just like the coconut) and is low GL. Still contains fructose, so use sparingly. Tastes similar to brown sugar.
- Stevia – in its natural form (a green powder), stevia is an excellent sweetener (if you can take the bitter aftertaste), but AVOID the processed white versions that the food industry has created.
- Dates (or date syrup) – a good alternative, especially in baking. Make pastes by soaking the fruits in water and blending.
- Blackstrap molasses – made by boiling sugar cane to remove much of the sugar and leave the remaining nutrient-rich syrup. A good alternative to golden syrup.
- Brown rice syrup – made by fermenting brown rice, it is lower GL than sugar and good for baking. Buy organic and gluten free.
- Yacon syrup – made without chemicals (so far!), yacon syrup is low GL and rich in probiotics – it might actually help with weight loss and diabetes!

Processed foods – foods with long lists of ingredients are to be avoided. As well as being packed full of sugar, salt and vegetable oils, they are usually full of food additives, preservatives, colours and flavourings that your body doesn't recognize and can interfere with hormone function.

Gluten-containing grains – this includes wheat, barley, rye and spelt. Not only do wheat products in particular raise insulin levels (some say quicker than pure sugar!), but also the gluten proteins can cause inflammation and stimulate your own immune system to attack your own tissue. One of the common targets is the thyroid gland (gluten sensitivity has been shown to be a major factor in Hashimoto's disease, an autoimmune thyroid disorder).

If you are having symptoms of any kind, I recommend you go gluten free for a few weeks. Gluten is at the root of many common symptoms and health conditions, and it's an easy thing to rule out if you're suffering. If you feel better at the end of your few weeks, try eating gluten again. If you suffer any bloating, headaches or fatigue you could have a gluten sensitivity (you will be among millions that do). Either get yourself tested, or avoid gluten forever more!

There are lots of great alternatives that you can switch to, such as quinoa, rice (brown or wild), buckwheat noodles and gluten-free pasta, but please be careful of the 'Gluten Free' aisle in the supermarket! Many of these foods may exclude gluten but they are heavily processed with lots of additives and chemicals – don't be duped into thinking they are healthy. Best to swap to alternative grains instead of gluten-free processed foods.

Foods that contain gluten

Wheat, rye, barley, spelt
Durum wheat
Kamut

Semolina
Bread and breaded or battered foods
Pasta and noodles
Soy sauce
Worcestershire sauce
Many flavoured crisps
Barley squashes
Beer, lager, stout, ales
Couscous
Bulgur wheat
Pies and pastries
Pizza
Cakes and biscuits
Dumplings and Yorkshire puddings
Sauces and gravies
Breakfast cereals
Muesli
Malt extract, syrup
Malt vinegar
Barley malt flavouring
Brewer's yeast
Edible starch

Trans-fats – many ready meals, spreads and packaged foods contain vegetable oils, as they are the cheapest oils to use (e.g. sunflower, safflower, canola or rapeseed). This type of fat can be highly INFLAMMATORY, raising cortisol in the body and increasing the risk of developing a chronic disease. Margarines and spreads are made from refined vegetable oil and are highly processed. Most ready meals, salad dressings, soups and other packaged goods are made with vegetable oils. That's why it's so important to look for real unprocessed foods and cook them yourself. You can use coconut oil, avocado oil, ghee, butter or animal fats for high heat cooking, olive oil for moderate heat cooking and good quality unrefined plant oils (olive, rapeseed, sesame) for dressings.

Alcohol – not only weakens resolve (you know that insane hunger after a few too many), but it also disrupts blood sugar and depletes nutrients, especially the B vitamins, which you need in plentiful supply to make your hormones happy. Alcohol is also a risk factor for cancers of the mouth, throat, colon, breast and liver. Try to give your liver a complete rest for a few weeks every year (dry January for me!), but if you can't do that, then some simple swaps can help; white wine to red (less sugar, more antioxidants), sugary mixers to soda water. And drink plenty of water between each drink and before you go to bed.

Foods to have in moderation

Limited dairy (milk, cheese, butter, cream, yoghurt)– you may want to experiment with excluding dairy for a few weeks. Not because it's inherently unhealthy (in fact organic dairy has a lot of essential nutrients), but because many people are lactose or casein intolerant without knowing it. Unless you have a severe reaction, this can be missed. If you want to, reintroduce afterwards and see how you feel. Try goats'/sheep's products first, then yoghurt, butter, milk. If you have any reaction, try lactose-free or A2 milk.

Ethnic lactose intolerance
Population studies seem to indicate that lactose intolerance is around 5–15% in Caucasian populations, but can be 70–100% in those of Asian and African descent.

Limited fruit – fruit is great in small quantities as the sugar contained comes with fibre and nutrients. But too much fruit sugar can spike your insulin, so I do recommend as a general rule limiting fruit to two pieces per day. Exceptions to this are berries and citrus fruits, as they are lower in sugar.

A word on SOY

Consumption of soy in Asia may be why women there have much lower incidences of hot flushes and other menopausal symptoms. However, the research on soy can be quite confusing. What I've found is that the majority of evidence shows that soy can be helpful for hormone balance, especially during menopause. And many studies even show that it's protective for breast cancer. It's important to avoid all non-organic and processed forms of soy, and stick to organic soy milk, yoghurt, tofu, edamame beans and fermented soy such as miso and tempeh. And avoid if you have any digestive reaction to it (it can be a common intolerance).

Foods for specific hormones

The general principles I have just covered will help you to balance your hormones and improve your well-being. These are foods that you can add to your diet to help with specific hormone imbalances.

Cortisol – if you have a cortisol imbalance, the actions in Step 2 will be very important for you. But your diet can also be really helpful:

- **Choose low GL (Glycaemic Load) foods** – e.g. sweet potatoes, brown or wild rice, quinoa, buckwheat, oats, pulses, beans, legumes, low sugar fruits – these will help to balance blood sugar, therefore reducing cortisol (which gets released when you have low blood sugar). See Resources for a low GL guide

- **B vitamins** – e.g. wholegrains, oats, meat, dairy, green veg, nuts, seeds – a range of B vitamins are needed for adrenal support
- **Vitamin C** – e.g. bell peppers, citrus fruits, broccoli – vitamin C helps to support adrenal reserve
- **Magnesium** – e.g. nuts, seeds, dark green leafy veg, dark chocolate – magnesium helps to relieve stress and increase relaxation
- **Avoid food stressors** – e.g. processed foods, sugar, alcohol, vegetable oils
- **Identify food sensitivities** – e.g. gluten, dairy, soy, eggs, corn
- **Eat protein and healthy fat at each meal** – not only will you feel fuller for longer, but also your blood sugar will be nice and stable
- **Sprinkle cinnamon on everything!** – cinnamon can help to balance blood sugar
- **Try a green protein smoothie for breakfast** – take a look at smoothies in Recipe section

Thyroid – thyroid hormones need good nutrient intake to function well. These include:

- **B vitamins** – e.g. wholegrains, oats, meat, dairy, green veg, nuts, seeds. B vitamins, especially B12 and B2, are needed to make thyroid hormones
- **Vitamin D** – from the sun – Vitamin D is needed to activate the thyroid receptor on the cell
- **Vitamin A** – e.g. liver, grass-fed butter, animal products – Vitamin A is also needed to activate thyroid receptors

- **Iron** – e.g. meat, poultry, fish, nuts, seeds, legumes, dried fruits, wholegrains – iron has a role in thyroid hormone synthesis and conversion
- **Selenium** – e.g. Brazil nuts, sesame and sunflower seeds, brown rice, meat, fish, eggs – selenium helps to convert T4 to T3
- **Zinc** – e.g. oysters, lamb, nuts, ginger, wholegrains, sardines – zinc is needed to produce TSH in the pituitary gland
- **Magnesium** – e.g. nuts, seeds, dark green leafy veg, dark chocolate – magnesium is also needed to produce TSH
- **Iodine** – e.g. fish and shellfish, sea vegetables (nori, dulse, kelp, wakame), eggs, dairy, meat, sea salt – iodine is needed to make your T4 hormone
- **Tyrosine** – e.g. chicken, turkey, fish, avocado, seeds, nuts, dairy, whey protein – tyrosine is the main amino acid in your T4 and T3 hormones
- **Omega 3 fats** – e.g. oily fish, flaxseeds, walnuts – Omega 3 fats help to protect thyroid cells
- **MCTs** (medium chain triglycerides) – coconut oil or liquid MCT oil – these fats help to boost metabolism
- **Avoid gluten** (especially if you have diagnosed hypothyroidism) – there are proven links between autoimmune thyroid conditions and coeliac disease
- **Avoid processed and non-organic soy** – e.g. soy isolate, soy 'meat', soy cheese etc as they might impair thyroid function

Oestrogen – certain dietary tweaks can help to regulate your oestrogen levels:

- **Phytoestrogens** – e.g. **organic soy, flaxseeds, lentils, chickpeas** – contain plant oestrogens that can help to balance your natural oestrogen levels

- **Fibre** – e.g. fruit, veg, wholegrains, nuts, seeds, beans, legumes, oats – can help to eliminate excess oestrogen
- **Go organic** – avoiding pesticides can reduce potential hormone disruption
- **Avoid mass-produced meat and dairy** – go organic and buy the best you can
- **Eat plenty of oily fish** – Omega 3 fats can help to reduce inflammation and help hormone balance

Francine's story

Menopausal bloat

Frances was 53 and fed up! She had all the classic signs of hormone imbalance due to menopause: fatigue, weight gain, hot flushes, insomnia and some digestive issues. She didn't want to go on HRT and wanted to try to deal with it naturally. Here's what she said after working with us:

'My weight had been creeping up year after year since my menopause, and I was suffering with low energy, poor sleep, hot flushes and digestive issues. Nicki got my hormones tested and put me on her programme. The first thing that improved was my sleep. What a difference that made! After two weeks I had lost 3kg without feeling hungry or deprived. After 30 days I had lost a total of 5kg, had got my energy back and the hot flushes and digestive issues had disappeared! I love my new healthy lifestyle and will never go back, thanks to Nicki's programme and support.'

- **Avoid alcohol** – alcohol can trigger hot flushes, but can also increase oestrogen levels – not good if you have either high or low levels
- **Eat your broccoli and cabbage** – cruciferous vegetables can help to get rid of excess oestrogen
- **Vitamin E** – e.g. almonds, sunflower seeds, olives, spinach, berries – can help to boost progesterone, reduce PMS and breast tenderness

Time-saving tips

One of the main issues many women have in their quest to eat more healthily is TIME.

I know how busy women are, especially if they're over 40 with family, work and other commitments. It's a big challenge juggling all the things we have to do!

And sometimes looking after yourself comes way down the list. That often means grabbing something quick and easy to eat, which may not be the healthiest option.

You can't get away from the fact that to feed your hormones well, you do need to choose fresh real food that isn't ready made or packaged (as much as possible).

But cooking from scratch can sometimes be time consuming. So here are my big time-saving tips:

- **Batch cooking** – bulk cooking a few dishes in advance (say on a weekend) and freezing into portions makes it super easy to heat something up during the week. One of my favourite things to do is to make a big bowl of quinoa tabbouleh (see Recipes) and keep it in the fridge for a quick lunch, snack or side dish. Just keep the olive oil dressing until you need it and it will stay fresh for days.

- **Upsize the recipes** – never just make one batch of anything. Double or treble the quantities, use as leftovers for lunch the next day or evening and freeze the rest. This includes side dishes and veg – they can all be added to salads or new dishes.

- Use some **'healthy processed foods'** – there is such a thing! I like to use ready cooked quinoa, rice and lentils to save time. Just make sure you use trusted brands and check the ingredients for any vegetable oils or additives.

- **Prepare your smoothie** the night before – throw your smoothie ingredients into your blender jug the night before (without the liquid) and pop into the fridge. Pour in your liquid in the morning – blend and go! Get yourself a cool blender bottle (PROMiXX do a good one) and you can give it a whizz before you drink it.

- **Prepare your lunch** – chop up your salad or lunch ingredients the night before, throw them together in the morning for a quick and easy packed lunch. If you have an oven or microwave at work, take in your precooked soup to warm up.

- **Get your shopping delivered** – if you're not set up for online shopping yet, this will save you loads of time. Have a 'favourites' list so you can quickly do your weekly shop. You can always top up during the week if you miss going to the store! My personal favourite online service is Ocado (their healthy range is second to none). I also like organic delivery boxes like Abel & Cole and Riverford for their fresh seasonal produce.

- **Stock up** on your store-cupboard essentials – these are the items you don't want to be running out of when you need to make a quick recipe – such as olive oil, coconut oil, spices, herbs, tahini, chickpeas, lentils, tomato passata, brown or wild rice, quinoa, nuts, seeds, and gluten-free pasta/noodles.

- **Get your family onboard!** If you have to cook something for yourself and then something else for your family, it's going to be tough. This eating plan is not a weird tasteless diet; it's all really delicious real foods! Try to get them onboard from the start – eating this way will benefit everyone. Or you can be a bit sneaky –they probably won't notice if you swap white rice for brown, or couscous for quinoa! (I swapped my kids' usual penne pasta for gluten-free brown rice pasta and no one said a word!)

Cooking methods

Even healthy foods can lose their nutrient value through poor cooking...

All fats have a smoke point, a temperature beyond which they change structure and become hazardous to health. For example, olive oil is safe up to 180°C: above this temperature (that includes most roasts and stir-fries) you should choose coconut oil, avocado oil, butter or other animal fats. If a recipe tells you to heat the oil first, just warm it: don't allow it to smoke or sizzle. Adding water or food to the pan keeps the temperature lower. If in doubt, it is much healthier to cook at lower temperatures. Never heat nut, vegetable and seed oils – use them only for dressings.

Be careful when cooking meat and fish to not burn or chargrill it. As soon as a food is browned or crisped, it can form unhealthy compounds called heterocyclic amines (HAs) and polycyclic aromatic hydrocarbons (PAHs), which have been linked to various cancers.

Much better to slow cook, poach or gently roast at lower temperatures.

When you cook vegetables, maximize the nutrients by steaming instead of boiling and keep the cooking time to a minimum. Eat some raw fruit and vegetables each day: a big mixed salad is perfect.

Timing: your secret weapon

So what you eat is incredibly important for your hormones. But WHEN you eat is also critical if you want to maximize results.

Are you a grazer?

'Eat every few hours' has been the mantra of virtually every dietician and nutritionist in the past 10 years. 'Got to keep your blood sugar stable...'

This is fine if you have hypoglycaemia or diabetes and need to eat to restore your blood sugar levels to safe amounts. Unfortunately this 'eat often' approach doesn't do much for the average woman. All it does is stimulate your pancreas to release more and more insulin to cope with all the times you are putting food into your mouth.

And we have taken this advice and become a nation of snackers. A whole industry has grown up around snacking that never existed in our grandparents' time. They lived on three good meals a day and snacking wasn't even a concept. I remember one of the first snack adverts on TV when I was little – 'a finger of fudge is just enough to give your kids a treat'. It took off and sparked the huge industry of snack foods that we now have.

Many experts believe that our snacking habit is a major factor behind the obesity epidemic. We know that when we eat food, our blood sugar rises and insulin stores it away as fat. Blood sugar levels usually give us energy for around three hours then the body starts to burn fat to keep us going. If we are constantly eating, we don't get the chance to burn fat – we just use up all the sugar stores.

So a gap of between 4–5 hours between meals is going to encourage your body to burn more fat. And if you get hungry, that's fine! Many of us have forgotten what that feels like in our 24/7 society with food everywhere. But it's totally normal and you're not going to starve! The feeling usually passes and you're OK again. In fact many of us think we're hungry when actually we just need water, or we're bored (or sad).

Having said that, if you're so hungry that you feel like killing someone, or you go dizzy or faint – then PLEASE EAT SOMETHING! Hypoglycaemia is rare but very serious, so listen to your body and be sensible.

Fasting

You may have heard about IF (intermittent fasting) and how it helps with weight loss and a host of other health markers, including ageing. While I can't argue with the science (and agree that it works well for a lot of people), I personally have serious concerns about this approach for women over 40, purely due to the hormone imbalances that they may have going on during this time that IF may not help with. It can upset your blood sugar and increase cortisol – not what we want!

In fact many women I have spoken to who have tried IF – either the 5:2 diet or the Alternate Day fast methods – have told me that they couldn't keep it going long term as it made them grumpy, tired and they got tempted to binge on their 'on' days on all the wrong foods.

But there is a much easier way to get the benefits of fasting without all the deprivation and calorie counting!

FAST WHILE YOU SLEEP!

You can get the same benefits of IF by giving your body an extended overnight fast – the ideal is 16 hours, but there are many benefits to gain in doing it for just 12 hours. Researchers in California fed one group of mice frequently throughout the day and night (equivalent to constant snacking or grazing), and the other group the same number of calories in an eight hour window. They were amazed when they found that the second group of mice were much healthier and much slimmer than the first group who all suffered from fatty liver and obesity.

The theory seems to be that while you are sleeping on an empty stomach, your body is better able to reset your metabolism and burn fat while you sleep. The reason is that the food you have eaten during the day has been stored as glycogen in your liver, and then slowly turned back into glucose during the night to keep your blood sugar stable and provide energy to your cells. If you run out of stored glucose (glycogen) your body will burn fat instead. So if you eat late, you won't run out of glycogen in time. You need to give your body enough rest time before you go to sleep, so that it can get to work burning fat a lot sooner. Makes sense, right?

And it's a lot easier than trying to burn it off at the gym for hours!

While 16 hours is ideal, it's not really very practical to do every night, especially if you want to eat out with friends or if you work late and need a later dinner. But 12-hour fasts are much easier and will have similar benefits. That means leaving 12 hours between dinner and breakfast every night. So if you have eaten at 8pm, then don't have your breakfast until 8am.

And then you can do a 16-hour fast when you are more able to (at weekends or on an evening when you're not going out or working late). That could mean dinner at 6pm, breakfast at 10am.

It's important not to eat or drink anything (apart from water) during these hours – no sneaking in a glass of wine or cup of tea!

SUMMARY

- Eat real foods!
- Fill half your plate with veg. Plenty of cruciferous.
- Enjoy fat – your hormones need it!
- Organic is best.
- Green and leafy rules. Coconut is king. Add nourishing superfoods.
- Make green protein smoothies. Stay hydrated.
- Batch cooking and upsizing saves you time in the kitchen.
- Cook with stable fats, dress with plant and seed oils.
- Don't graze. Eat three good meals a day. Fast overnight.

STEP 2 – REST

Stress management

As you saw in Chapter 3, the impact of stress on your general health and hormones is huge. Elevated stress hormones over time can raise blood pressure, increase fat stores, decrease energy, suppress immunity, impair digestion and sex hormone function. All of this can cause PMS, digestive issues, frequent infections, insomnia, fertility problems, depression, fat around the middle, fatigue, brain fog, mood swings and higher risk of heart disease and diabetes.

This is serious. If you don't prioritize stress management in your life, your chances of a good healthy old age are pretty slim... (even if you have the best diet in the world!).

And you could be heading for adrenal fatigue; wiped out and exhausted. That's what can happen if you let chronic stress go on for too long.

Imagine you have a Stress Bucket

All your different types of stress feed into the bucket; work stress, families, financial worries, emotions, relationships, poor diet, lack of sleep, chemicals and more. Some might be more than others, but they all accumulate. It gets full pretty quickly. And it keeps filling up on a daily basis. The holes in the bucket represent your coping mechanisms, allowing your stresses to dissipate and keeping your bucket from overflowing.

But when you're too stressed or your coping mechanisms aren't enough, your bucket can overflow and your body can start to break down, very gradually, leaving you at increased risk of exhaustion and chronic health conditions.

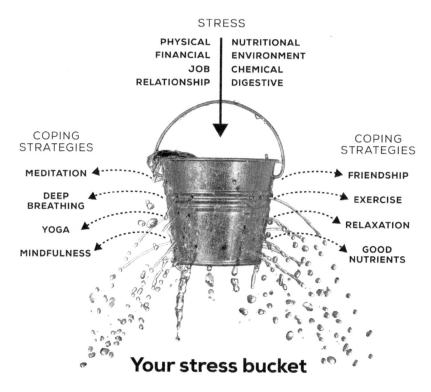

Your stress bucket

Too much stress going in and not enough coping strategies will cause the bucket to overflow and health starts to suffer

I know we can't avoid stress, that's just part of modern life. But we do have control over how much rest and relaxation we get, and that allows the body to recover and cope with whatever life throws at us. (If you are a high achiever type, take note that recent studies have shown that the more rest you get and the fewer hours you work, the more productive you are!)

So how do you manage your stress?

1. Reduce your obvious stressors
Stress is not always obvious. You will be aware of the obvious things like work, family, relationships, traffic, bereavement, etc.

But often your stress is deep-seated and underlying (so much so that you don't know it's there!).

- Identify your obvious stressors. Go through the list of potential sources of stress listed in Chapter 3 and tick any that may be a problem for you.
- Put a plan in place to reduce or eliminate them. You may need some expert help to do this, and it may take some time, but if you don't go for the source, you will always be dealing with the consequences.
- Establish and protect your boundaries – learn to say NO more often. Women are natural people pleasers and tend to take on too much. Go through your calendar and cancel things you really don't want to do. It's very liberating!

De-stress your diet
Follow the principles in Step 1 (Eat) to take the potential stressors out of your diet. And don't follow any more DIETS – they are stressful!

De-stress your environment
Follow the principles in Step 3 (Cleanse) to minimize your exposure to potential chemical stressors.

De-stress your emotions
If your source of stress is coming from your emotions, you will need to get specialist help to deal with it. Whether it's a past trauma, low self-esteem, relationship issues, feelings of loneliness, grief or anger, or something else, if you don't address it, it will always be a source of stress for you whatever you do to be healthy in other areas.

2. Switch off more
Counteract your fight or flight response by switching on your parasympathetic nervous system (rest and repair mode). To do this, you need to slow right down:

- **Breathing** – deep breathing from your belly, helps to reset your stress hormones, which helps with weight loss, anxiety, mood and brain function! With one hand on your belly, inhale through the nose to a count of five, pushing your belly up and breathing into the lower part of your lungs. As you breathe out for five, slowly feel your belly fall. Do this 10 times, once or twice a day, or whenever you feel stressed.
- **Mindfulness** – silencing the chatter in your mind and being 'mindful' (concentrating on the task in hand, being present) – has huge benefits for your overall health. Try mindful eating – concentrate fully and notice the look, texture, smell and taste of your food as you are eating. This will not only slow you down and fill you up quicker, but also will really relax you and make your food taste great! You can also try mindful walking, driving, queuing, travelling on a train, brushing teeth, listening, the opportunities are endless!
- **Yoga** – for me yoga is a double whammy – great exercise and a huge stress reducer. The trick is to find a class that suits you. There are many styles and teachers, so classes vary hugely. You may hate one and love another. So stick with the search until you find one you love.
- **Nature** – getting outside into nature, getting some sun if you can, going for a walk – all great for reducing cortisol levels.
- **Hobbies** – music, relaxation tapes, cooking, Scrabble, gardening – whatever you love doing will help you relax.
- **Reading** – one of the easiest and fastest ways to reduce stress (and a great one to make you sleepy). Just six minutes has been shown to be effective.
- **Massage** – sounds like a luxury? Having a 15-minute massage once a week has actually been shown to reduce

cortisol, lower blood pressure and increase serotonin and dopamine.

- **Be sociable** – having good friends and a support network is a huge stress reliever. Note the 'good' friends bit – people that bring you down and drain you are definitely not going to help your cortisol levels – dump them if you can, seriously.
- **Laughter** – seeing a funny film or TV show, or being with someone who makes you laugh is a great way to de-stress – scientifically proven!
- **Take your holidays!** – so many of you are working way too hard, long hours, weekends and some of you are not even taking your holiday allowance! If that's the only time you switch off, then make sure you book your time off work in advance and stick to it. You don't have to go away on holiday, just take a break from your work environment (and emails!).
- **Try a total digital detox** – just for one day a week (it's hard I know!) but so good to give your system a break.
- **Get sexy** – while low libido can be an issue during the perimenopausal years, sex is incredibly good for your cortisol levels. Oxytocin is released during sex (especially during orgasm) and this reduces stress and anxiety, boosts natural endorphins and helps you sleep. If dryness is an issue, try a natural lubricant (or discuss bio-identical vaginal gels, creams or pessaries with your doctor).
- **Get 'grounded'** – have you heard of earthing? It's when your body is in contact with the ground – either barefoot outdoors or on an earthing surface inside. Doesn't it feel good when you're walking barefoot in the sand or on grass (think summer holiday, not mid UK winter!!)? The surface of the earth has a lot of free electrons that

get transferred to your skin when you're in contact with it. Scientific studies are showing huge benefits of doing this regularly, especially in the areas of stress, pain management, cardiovascular health and sleep.

There are lots of options and I know it's not easy to make relaxation a priority if your life is busy, but you need to find whatever it is that works for you and make it part of your routine – no excuses. List 10 activities that make you happy or calm and make sure you do one every day.

3. Sleep
So you saw in Chapter 4 how stress and poor sleep are linked, and the consequences of lack of sleep on your hormones and your risk of long-term health issues. Sleeping is your natural anti-stress remedy. And of course it's more difficult when you're stressed!

But easier said than done, right? The more you know how important sleep is, the more you're going to stress about not getting enough, and the less sleep you get…

Tips to get a good night's sleep

- **Darkness** – make sure the room is totally dark – artificial light (especially the blue light from electronics) interferes with your production of melatonin, the sleep hormone. Get some blackout blinds and cover any electronic lights from your alarm clock, phone, TV or laptop. If for any reason you can't get rid of all light, then use an eye mask. If you have to use your laptop, tablet or phone, try wearing blue light blocking glasses like BluBlockers.
- **Go to bed earlier** – research has shown that the hours before midnight are more restorative. During sleep we have several cycles of REM and deeper non-REM sleep. Between 11pm and 3am, we have more cycles of deeper

non-REM sleep, and that is when the body does more of its repair work. So try to get to bed before 11pm every night.

- **Get off the gadgets**! Your brain will be overstimulated and it will be hard to switch off if you're on your laptop, phone or tablet at night. Try not to keep them in your bedroom overnight. If left on, the electromagnetic frequencies they emit can interfere with your melatonin production.

- **Balance your blood sugar** – avoid quick release carbohydrates (e.g. white bread, potatoes, sugar, processed foods), which put you on the blood sugar roller coaster. Some people do well on eating at least three hours before bed. Others do well on having a small low GL snack just before bed (like some nuts or seeds).

- **Limit your caffeine** – I love my coffee, but I can't drink it after lunchtime without it affecting my sleep. We all have different tolerance levels to caffeine, and as we age our tolerance can decrease. For some people, it can take longer for caffeine to clear from the body, so if you have problems sleeping, avoid it for a week and see what happens. Caffeine is also a diuretic so you may find you don't have to get up at night if you eliminate it.

- **Exercise** – as well as boosting endorphins, being physically tired can result in more relaxing sleep at night.

- **Have a soak** – a regular warm bath helps to soothe muscles and reduce stress. Add some Epsom salts for your magnesium (one cup poured into warm water) and enjoy a good soak for about 20 minutes.

- **Magnesium** is the calming mineral – essential for relaxing nerves and muscles. If you prefer a shower to a bath, you can get your magnesium in supplement form (spray, oil, tablet, powder). See Chapter 11 for more information.

- **Herbal teas** – try a calming herbal tea before bed. There are many night time formulas out there. Pukka Night Time is one of my favourites.
- **Banana tea** – banana peel has a very high magnesium content. You can't eat it, but you can boil the skin for five minutes in water, cool it down and drink the flavoured water before bed.
- **Pick up a book** – reading reduces cortisol, so naturally makes you more relaxed and sleepy.
- **Calm your mind** – going over and over things that have happened or are planned in the future can stop anyone sleeping. Best to write it all down to get it out of your head and try a relaxation or meditation App or CD.
- **No news** – watching the news, a thriller or a scary film before bed can stress you out, so try to avoid.
- **Avoid alcohol** 4–6 hours before bed – a drink is great for getting you off to sleep initially, but as the alcohol wears off it has a stimulatory effect at about 3am! It may be hard to get back to sleep afterwards.

4. Restore nutrients

The adrenal glands use up a lot of nutrients to keep pumping out stress hormones. The main ones are:

- B vitamins – found in oats, nuts, seeds, leafy veg, organic meat, fish, dairy
- Vitamin C – eat a rainbow of fruit and veg, especially bell peppers, kiwi fruit, citrus fruit, green leafy veg
- Magnesium – dark green leafy veg, nuts, seeds, brown rice, beans, avocado, dark chocolate, many fruits and veggies (you can also absorb it from Epsom salts baths or magnesium oil)

5. Supplement

In therapeutic doses, supplements can work very quickly to restore adrenal balance (<u>always check with your doctor or health practitioner before starting any new supplements</u>):

- A good quality B complex – especially B5 and B6
- Vitamin C
- Magnesium (citrate or glycinate are better absorbed forms)
- Phosphatidylserine – a brain phospholipid that can help to boost dopamine and reduce cortisol
- Herbal adaptogens – eg rhodiola, ashwagandha, holy basil, lemon balm, liquorice root – can all help to balance cortisol levels

Ommmmm… the benefits of meditation

What do you think of when you hear the word 'meditation'? Super stretchy people sitting cross-legged chanting?

Well, meditation doesn't have to be like that. How about we call it 'sitting quietly time'? How often in your day do you just sit and do nothing? Or it can just be a moment of mindfulness, standing on a train or walking in a park. Just a few minutes a day of clearing your mind of clutter can make all the difference.

If you haven't tried it, I urge you to give it a go. You don't have to sit cross-legged on the floor, just sit comfortably on a chair, you need to be upright though with your back straight, feet on the floor. Sit for 10 minutes quietly with your eyes closed. You can listen to a guided meditation (plenty on YouTube), or you can just focus on your breathing, or you can listen to sounds. The idea is to be in the present moment. This switches you into relaxation mode, turns off your cortisol and sends a clear message to the brain that you are not in danger, no need for all those stress hormones, no need to hang on to fat and give you cravings.

These are the things meditation has been shown to help with:

- Lowering your heart rate and reducing your blood pressure
- Reducing stress hormones (cortisol and adrenaline), switching on our parasympathetic nervous system – the rest and repair function
- Improving your mood
- Boosting creativity
- Relieving pain
- Reducing anxiety
- Boosting immunity
- Increasing fertility and sex drive
- Reducing IBS symptoms
- Reducing inflammation
- Improving sleep
- Reducing binge and emotional eating, promoting weight loss
- Reducing your risk of cancer and heart disease

And if you're worried that you're not 'doing it properly', you might want to read Russell Simmon's book *Success Through Stillness*. He says the misconception that often stops people:

'is the belief that they're not "good" at meditating. These people make the effort to sit down and meditate but then don't stick with the practice because they feel like they're "doing it wrong" or somehow aren't having the same experience that "real" meditators do. Meditation does not mean the absence of thoughts.

Meditation does not mean going into a trance.

Meditation does not mean forgetting who or where you are.

If you're worrying that you're not "doing it right" because none of those things happen when you meditate, then please stop worrying.'

SUMMARY

- Chill out. Relax. Breathe deeply.
- Sleep well.
- Don't be a stress junkie. Be present.
- Take regular breaks from technology.
- Meditate or be still every day.
- Do more of what you enjoy.
- Say NO more often!
- Support your adrenals.

STEP 3 – CLEANSE

In Chapter 4 you saw how your hormones are under constant attack from toxins in your environment. They can act as a major stress on the body and put pressure on your adrenal organs as well as your liver and gut. This can increase cortisol levels, disrupt thyroid function, increase oestrogen levels and really mess up your hormone balance.

Unless you live in some kind of bubble, you are exposed to these toxins every day. You can't avoid them and indeed your own body produces toxins from your metabolic processes. We are designed to deal with our own internal waste products and some limited toxins from our environment, but we have never been exposed to so many different toxins before and there is plenty of evidence that it is seriously affecting our health.

Even though many of these individual chemicals have been proved 'safe', we still don't know about the cumulative effect of these substances. While more studies are definitely needed, it seems the sensible option would be to reduce your chemical exposure wherever possible. It might seem daunting at first, but there are actually a lot of simple things you can do to live a more natural life and support your liver.

Detoxing your world

Detoxing has become a huge money spinner with a zillion products on the shelves promising to clean us out and solve all our problems. But you don't need to live on cabbage soup and lemons to detox yourself!

All you need is to limit your exposure to the toxins, and support your own detoxification systems (your gut and liver) – you don't need any fancy potions, starvation diets or complicated programmes.

Clean environment

If you live in the city, you will have to deal with pollution in the air. If you live in the countryside, you don't escape toxic air – you may live close to an agricultural farm where pesticides are used, residues of which can drift in the air and spread. If you smoke or hang around with smokers, or you work in a chemical environment (hair/nail salon, dry cleaners, factory, aeroplane, etc) – you are more exposed than most and will need to take steps to protect yourself.

Stick with me; it's not all doom and gloom! Here are some things you can do to reduce your exposure:

- Avoid cigarette smoke
- Use indoor plants to help filter the air (peace lilies and aloe vera plants are my favourites)
- Planting trees outside helps to absorb pollution from busy roads
- Switch from carpet to wooden floors
- If you have to have something dry-cleaned, hang it out to air before wearing it
- Air ionizers can help remove indoor pollutants

If you work in a chemical-heavy environment, awareness is key. If you have health problems you might need to think about whether you can change your job. If this isn't possible, think about some form of protection like breathing masks, especially if you are inhaling chemicals directly.

Clean products

Our modern world has produced over 84,000 known chemicals that are used in almost every product that we buy for our homes, gardens, personal care, cars and pets.

We either breathe these chemicals in or we put them on our skins to absorb straight into our bloodstream.

Swap to organic, natural products for your home, skin and hair – have a look at online stores like Big Green Smile and Ethical Superstore.

And type your products into the handy new App 'Think Dirty', which checks the ingredients and rates them out of 10.

- Swap to natural cleaning products
- Use essential oils for fragrance
- Swap to natural toiletries
- Swap to natural cosmetics
- Use non-fluoride toothpaste
- Use natural deodorant
- Swap to natural sunscreen
- Avoid weedkillers and other garden chemicals
- Swap to non-toxic pet flea treatments
- Limit your dry cleaning
- Use natural hair colourants (or be a Silver Sister!)
- Use glass, cast iron, ceramic or steel cookware instead of Teflon and aluminium
- Use paper or non-PVC wrap instead of cling film

Tampons

We love the convenience of using tampons but that convenience can come at a price. Tampons allow bacteria to breed and this can cause problems. Most commercial tampons contain rayon, which makes them highly absorbent. The fibres in rayon not only bring oxygen into the vagina (a non-oxygen environment) which can encourage bacteria to grow, but the fibres can also get left behind, providing a breeding ground for toxins and a risk of toxic shock syndrome (TSS). This is where toxins from the vagina get into your bloodstream and cause severe infection.

The materials used in tampon manufacture are also bleached white with chlorine, releasing by-products called dioxins. Dioxins are harmful carcinogens and EDCs (endocrine disrupting chemicals). Not to mention the environmental damage from thousands of tampons clogging up our sewage and landfills!

Luckily we have new and innovative products that we can switch to. Ever heard of the Mooncup? It's a reusable silicone cup that sits inside the vagina. It's easy to use and totally safe. You do have to get intimate with the contents of your period but, if you can get over that, it's a great alternative to tampons. If you can't face that, then look for organic cotton tampons that are much kinder to you and the environment.

BPA

How to avoid over-exposure:

- Use glass, ceramic or stainless steel bottles and food containers. I am loving the range of funky glass water bottles you can get now.
- Don't ever put plastic containers in the microwave – heating can cause the BPA to leach out into the food.
- Don't wrap fatty foods like cheese in cling film – because BPA is lipophilic (fat loving), these foods can absorb it from the wrap. Try paper wraps or non-PVC wrap.
- Avoid canned foods (especially acidic foods like tomatoes), choose glass or paper carton packaging.

Clean water

You saw what some tap waters can contain in Chapter 4. Why not drink filtered or bottled water to be on the safe side? I know not all bottled waters are good, and there's the plastic and environment to consider. Water filter jugs now come in glass, or you can have a filter fitted to your tap or to the pipe coming in to your house (often called 'whole house filters'). Filters vary, so do some research. I like the reverse osmosis system with a remineralizer, although I am still saving up for mine!

Clean diet

You don't need to go on some crazy 'detox' regime to clean out your system. You just need to support your own body's detoxification processes.

- Eat organic to avoid petrochemicals, herbicides, pesticides, antibiotics and hormones.
- Increase your vegetable intake – cruciferous vegetables like broccoli, cauliflower, cabbage, green leafy veg and salads – help the liver detoxify, and contain indole-3-carbinol, a substance that helps metabolize and eliminate oestrogen.
- Increase sulphur-containing foods – e.g. eggs, garlic, leeks, onions – to help with detoxification.
- Avoid processed foods – eat whole real foods where possible.
- Eat more fibre – having regular bowel movements helps your body detoxify. Fibre also helps to bind excess oestrogen and eliminate it.
- Increase your probiotics – beneficial gut bacteria can help your detoxification processes.
- Try to limit cooking food at high temperatures (BBQ, frying, roasting) as this can produce toxic by-products.

Switch to slow cooking or low temperature cooking, especially for meats.

- Eat clean fish – wild (not farmed), line-caught or organic.
- Watch your caffeine and alcohol intake. Detoxing these two takes up a lot of the liver's resources, so give your liver a well-earned rest (if that seems too hard, remember the 80/20 rule!).

Up your antioxidants! Increasing your intake of vitamins A, E, C, selenium and zinc can help prevent too many free radicals forming (the ones that speed up ageing!) and help your liver detoxification processes:

- Vitamin A – liver, grass-fed meat, butter, orange/red vegetables
- Vitamin C – peppers, broccoli, berries, green leafy veg, fruits
- Vitamin E – nuts, seeds, avocados, oily fish
- Selenium – seeds, Brazil nuts, tuna, cabbage
- Zinc – seafood, grass-fed meat, almonds, pumpkin seeds

Other ways to help your body to DETOX:

- Epsom salts baths – these salts are made from magnesium sulphate and when you soak your body in a bath containing a handful of them, your skin absorbs the magnesium, helping to relax your muscles, improve circulation and aid the delivery of nutrients and elimination of waste. The sulphur helps support the liver's detoxification pathways too.
- Sweating is a great way to get rid of toxins. The skin is one of your most important detoxification organs. Exercise, saunas, steam rooms – try anything that gets your sweat dripping.

- Dry skin brushing – brushing your skin upwards towards your heart, helps to mobilize the lymphatic drainage system, getting rid of toxins.
- Massage, yoga, deep breathing – all help with circulation and elimination of waste.

Foods to support your liver

- Cruciferous veg – e.g. broccoli, cauliflower, cabbage, sprouts, watercress, kale, rocket, bok choy, collard greens, Brussels sprouts – help to detoxify oestrogen
- Garlic, eggs, leeks, onions for good sulphur content
- Green tea – a potent antioxidant
- Fresh vegetable juices including carrots, celery, coriander, beetroot, parsley, and ginger – liver-supporting nutrients and antioxidants
- Herbal teas containing a mixture of liver supporting herbs – burdock root, dandelion root, ginger root, liquorice root, sarsaparilla root, cardamom seeds, cinnamon bark and other herbs
- Artichokes – help stimulate bile flow
- Flaxseeds (or linseeds) for oestrogen regulation
- Citrus peels, caraway and dill oil (they contain limonene)
- Bioflavonoids in grapes, berries and citrus fruits
- Celery to increase the flow of urine and aid in detoxification
- Coriander (cilantro), which may help remove heavy metals
- Rosemary, which has carnosol, a potent booster of detoxification enzymes
- Turmeric for its antioxidant and anti-inflammatory action

What about juice diets?

I love juicing, there's nothing better than giving your body a huge dose of TLC – the nutrients from a fresh vegetable juice go straight into your cells for a big nourishment hit. Your digestion also gets a bit of a break too – it doesn't have to do much work, so you are likely to feel much more energetic. And great if you have any digestion problems.

BUT juices don't contain any fibre, protein or fat. You need all of these for your liver and gut to work efficiently, to balance your blood sugar and for absorption of the fat-soluble vitamins A, D, E and K.

So if you are doing a juice-only programme, make sure you are adding in some protein (protein powder, nuts, seeds, spirulina) and some **healthy fat** (avocado, nuts, seeds, coconut oil/milk). And don't use fruits for juicing; you'll just get a huge hit of sugar straight into the blood. Just juice the vegetables, then put them in the blender with your other ingredients to make a super nutritious juice-based smoothie.

SUMMARY

- Gradually swap your household products to natural non-toxic brands
- Filter your water
- Limit caffeine and alcohol
- Eat organic
- Up your antioxidants and cruciferous veg
- Sweating, Epsom salts baths and dry brushing all help with detoxification

STEP 4 – MOVE

In Chapter 4, we looked at how your lifestyle (or how much you move) affects your hormone balance. Too much sitting and too little moving in general is definitely a hormone disruptor, but equally too MUCH exercise can also be a bad thing.

Physical activity is so important for hormones. It can:

- increase circulation – improving delivery of nutrients and oxygen to cells
- increase HDL (good) cholesterol
- support detoxification and elimination of waste material
- support bone health
- improve your mood by increasing endorphins
- improve immunity – better lymphatic circulation will help immune function
- reduce stress – although excessive exercise can increase cortisol, moderate exercise can reduce stress levels and help you sleep
- stimulate fat burning and increase energy
- improve lung capacity, increasing oxygen levels and reducing stress
- strengthen your heart and blood vessels
- improve your sex drive

All in all it can add an extra seven years to your life expectancy! Now that's an incentive…

And of course it's good for your hormones. Without activity, your muscles waste away, your fat stores go up, your circulation stagnates and you are at much higher risk of serious disease.

But finding the right 'Goldilocks' amount for you is the secret.

Top 5 activities for happy hormones

1. Reduce sitting time

Most of us sit for far too long, but it just takes a few habit changes to make it less damaging to your health (and hormones). Research even shows getting up and walking around for two minutes out of every hour can increase your lifespan by 33%, compared to those who do not.

Here are some other ideas:

- walk and talk – instead of that coffee shop meet up, arrange a walking meeting
- mobile walking – when you're on your mobile phone, get up and walk with it
- set an alarm – set your phone or computer to ping at you every hour to remind you to get up and take a quick break (check out Apps like Time Out and BreakTime)
- if you work from home, invest in a standing desk or Walkstation
- get a Fitbit or pedometer to track your steps – join a group for extra motivation
- make some new rules – always use stairs instead of lifts, walk up every escalator, park further away from where you need to be, get off the train or bus a stop earlier, do some squats while you are watching TV (or when the ads are on) – any excuse to move more!

2. Walking

I'm a huge fan of walking. It's easy to do, cheap (no gym membership or equipment involved) and it has huge benefits. AND if you go outside into nature, you get the added benefits of improved mood and feeling calmer. Just 30 minutes a day has been shown to:

- reduce risk of heart disease
- improve blood pressure
- improve blood sugar balance
- lower the risk of obesity
- reduce your risk of breast and colon cancer
- enhance mental well-being
- reduce your risk of type 2 diabetes
- reduce your risk of osteoporosis

If you need motivation to go out for a walk, join a local group or get yourself a dog!

3. HIIT – fast track your exercise routine

What if I told you that you could get the same benefits (actually even more benefits) from exercise in a fraction of the time it takes you currently? Instead of two to three trips to the gym every week (or two to three runs) you could exercise for just 15 minutes two or three times a week?

HIIT – high intensity interval training has been shown to burn fat more effectively than aerobic exercise. As well as strengthening your lungs and heart, it also increases human growth hormone (HGH), the hormone that is abundant when you are young, making you healthy and strong, but declines rapidly as you age. Another huge advantage is that HIIT improves insulin sensitivity, a great result for your waistline and reducing your risk of serious disease. And recent research has shown that HIIT can not only suppress your appetite but it can prolong your fat burning for many hours after your workout!

You can choose how to do HIIT: sprinting, cycling, swimming, walking and circuit training are all good ways to start. The best thing about it is that you only have to set aside 15 minutes, two or three times a week, to have a dramatic effect on your health – and you don't need to go to the gym. You can get on an exercise bike, run up and down stairs, skip, sprint with the dog – anything that gets your heart (and lungs) racing.

Instructions
1. Warm up for 3 minutes (a gentle jog, or some squats/push ups)
2. Push yourself as hard as you can for 30 seconds, until you are gasping for breath and have to stop
3. Then rest for 60 seconds
4. Repeat seven more times

So that's a total of eight bursts of 30 seconds – four minutes in total. With the rest and warm-up time, it comes to just over 14 minutes for your whole workout. Not only is it quicker than running for an hour, but you will continue to reap the benefits for longer.

(Don't attempt HIIT training if you are exhausted, unfit or overly stressed as it could make things worse.)

4. Resistance and weights
Muscle mass declines as you age (at a rapid rate if you don't do any strength training!). The more muscle you have the more calories you burn, day and night, reducing your fat stores. High cortisol has a negative effect on muscle mass, so building muscle is really important if you're overstressed. Your fat:muscle ratio is what you are aiming to improve (note – you may not see as much weight loss if you are increasing muscle to fat). Strength training also lowers your risk of osteoporosis, which is a risk factor during and after menopause.

Weight training doesn't mean turning into Arnie in the gym! A set of weights at home will do the trick, or you can go outside and use a park bench if that's your preference.

5. Yoga and Pilates
Yoga and Pilates have so many benefits. They improve flexibility, strength, posture, stress and mood. They are the ultimate anti-ageing activities!

When I do yoga, I am so focused on the pose I am trying to hold (and remembering to breathe!) that it is impossible for me to think about anything else. This forces me to be present (not lingering on the morning's stresses or trying to plan the evening's dinner). Being mindful or fully present is so difficult in our busy lives that taking the time to do it, plus strengthening your body at the same time, is a great thing to do. There are so many different types of yoga that it can be confusing at first. My advice would be to try different classes until you find one you love. It might take a while, but persevere. Once you find the one, it will be true love I promise!

I haven't included endurance-type cardio in this list, not because there's anything wrong with it (there are lots of benefits to cardio work!), but it just doesn't make my top five for hormone balancing after 40. If you run long distances, that's fine, as long as you have the energy for it, you don't get regular injuries and you're not suffering from adrenal fatigue.

<u>Please be careful if you have a health condition or haven't tried any of this before. Check with your doctor before undertaking any new exercise programme.</u>

SUMMARY

- Sit less, move more – take regular breaks
- Walking is a winner
- HIIT is for fast track fat burning
- Focus on muscle maintenance
- Yoga and Pilates tick all the boxes
- Over-exercising will stress your body and encourage fat storing

Love your gut!

We saw in Chapter 6 how important your gut health is to your hormone health. As well as following Step 1 of the Happy Hormone Code and eliminating foods that can harm your gut lining (and therefore prevent you absorbing all the nutrients from your new healthy diet!), there are some specific gut-friendly things you can start doing straight away:

- **Eat slowly!** Take your time and chew properly – you start digesting with the saliva in your mouth (the cephalic phase of digestion). The more work you do here, the less work the rest of your system has to do.
- **Don't graze;** try to limit snacking (unless you are hypoglycaemic). Eating three good meals a day gives the digestive system time to rest in between.
- **Take a sip of apple cider vinegar before meals** – this has been shown to help increase stomach acid levels and aid digestion.
- **Reduce your stress levels** – cortisol can impair stomach acid production and reduce your defences against toxins and microbes. This can imbalance your gut flora (not enough good bacteria), allow toxins through the gut wall and prevent absorption of nutrients.
- **Remove food triggers** – if you follow Step 1 of the Happy Hormone Code, then you will be limiting three of the most common foods that can cause a reaction (gluten, dairy, soy). But if you suspect you may have a food intolerance to something else, then go without it for at least three weeks, then reintroduce and see if you get a reaction.
- **Watch your medications** – take them if they are essential of course, but don't just pop a painkiller or take antibiotics

if they are not totally necessary. Medications can irritate the gut lining and impact the delicate balance of your gut flora.

- **Don't overdo the indigestion tablets**! If you suffer from acid reflux or heartburn, it is most likely due to a weak valve letting the contents of your stomach into your oesophagus, and NOT due to too much acid. Stomach acid is vital to digest protein, absorb vitamin B12 and kill any microbes you eat. When you take antacids over a long period of time, it can seriously reduce your acid levels, compromising your digestion.
- **Eat plenty of fibre** – especially soluble fibre found in fruit and veg, nuts, seeds, pulses (flaxseeds are a great source). Fibre helps keep food moving through your system, taking toxins with it (and especially helps keep oestrogen levels down).
- **Eat fermented foods** – full of probiotics, fermented foods such as sauerkraut, live yoghurt, miso, kefir and kombucha help to repopulate the good bacteria.
- **Go easy on the alcohol!** – It can irritate the gut lining and alter your gut flora balance.
- **Check for infection** – get yourself tested if you suffer from IBS or other digestive issues (bloating, gas, constipation, diarrhoea, indigestion). Contact us for more info (www.happyhormonesforlife.com/contact).
- **Make your own meat stocks** (or bone broth) – stock or broth from simmering bones and vegetables for hours contains gelatine, which is really good for your gut. It also has lots of nutrients that nourish the gut lining, supporting the barrier against toxins. Check out the Recipes section for my easy chicken stock.

Mindful eating

1. **Start gradually** – if this is new to you, it's best to start with one meal or snack each day and commit to mindful eating just once a day.
2. **Switch off** – it's really difficult to focus on eating if you're doing other things. Turn off your phone and laptop. Set aside time for eating without any distractions. Enjoy some quiet time, just you and your food.
3. **Cook or prepare from scratch** – if you're ripping off the plastic and diving in, you are not giving yourself time for that crucial cephalic phase of digestion. By preparing food yourself (even if it's throwing a salad together), you are not only eating more healthily but you are also improving your digestion and absorption processes. Cooking can also be very relaxing, so you are helping to switch off your stress response.
4. **Start small** – if you're eating a snack, lay it out in small portions. If you're eating a meal, use a knife and fork to cut it into bite-sized chunks to eat one at a time.
5. **Wait before eating!** Just take a few moments to look and appreciate what you're about to eat; notice the colour, shape, texture. If you're reaching into the fridge or cupboard for a snack, stop and ask yourself 'am I really hungry?'
6. **Notice each mouthful**. As you put the food into your mouth, pay close attention to the sensations – taste, texture, crunch, how it feels as you chew. If you're with others, ask them how it tastes, and share your observations.
7. **Chew!** Make sure you chew your mouthful thoroughly – enough to make it into a liquid before swallowing. This will really help your digestion.

8. **Finish your mouthful** before eating any more – how many times do we take the next mouthful while we're still chewing the first one? Wait until you have swallowed before taking the next bite. It might help to put your cutlery down between mouthfuls.
9. **Stop eating** when you feel 80% full – by eating mindfully, you should feel full a lot quicker. Try to stop eating when you start getting those satiety messages, not when the plate is empty!
10. **Be grateful** – take a moment to feel some gratitude for the food you've just eaten. How often do we take for granted that we have such amazing food available to us?

It can take a long time to get your digestive system fully back to normal. You may need to work with a qualified health practitioner to get properly tested and started on a gut repair protocol.

Naomi's story

Brain fog

Naomi was a successful 47-year-old business owner (and mum) at the end of her tether. She was exhausted and couldn't think straight any more. It was really affecting her life. She was struggling to make decisions in her business, she couldn't concentrate on anything and she was forgetting her client's names! She thought it might be her hormones so came to see us to try to find some answers. At the end of the programme, this is what she had to say:

'I put my growing fatigue and brain fog down to my hormones and being a busy business owner and mum. But when we ran some tests, we discovered it was a candida infection that was to blame! With Nicki's support, and a really effective diet and supplement programme, I have now regained control over my life. I'm really grateful for her advice!'

Summary

- Eat slowly and chew thoroughly
- Get more fibre and fermented foods into your diet
- Reduce stress to support digestion
- Check for underlying infections

Get your vitamin D

We saw in Chapter 4 how deficient we all are in vitamin D, for obvious reasons if you live in the UK!

Where do we get it from?

The main source of vitamin D is from direct sunlight, so unless you're holidaying in the Caribbean every few weeks during the winter months, you are likely going to be deficient. According to UK Government guidelines, we only get enough sunlight to make vitamin D between mid May and September. You can get small amounts from animal foods, such as egg yolks, meat, oily fish and dairy, but it's not enough to keep your levels in the optimal range.

You can get a good 10,000iu of vitamin D from exposure to direct sunlight in 10–20 minutes (without sun cream). The skin absorbs the UVB radiation from the sun, converts it to vitamin D3, then the liver and kidneys transform it again into the active form $(1,25(OH)_2D)$ to do its work.

If you are at risk of not getting enough vitamin D from either lack of sunshine, cultural reasons, darker skin type, kidney or liver conditions, pregnancy, excess stress, obesity or genetics, then you will need to supplement.

How do you know how much you need?

You need to get your levels tested to properly determine how much you need to supplement:

- ask your doctor for a test
- order a home test kit. In the UK, this is the one I recommend: http://www.vitamindtest.org.uk

Reference range UK

Status	Blood level
Deficient	< 25 nmol
Insufficient	25–50 nmol
Adequate	50–75 nmol
Optimal	>75 nmol

Like anything, toxicity is possible if you take too much for a long period of time, but experts say that occurrences are very rare and many high dose supplement protocols have been undertaken with no adverse effects.

The current daily recommendation for vitamin D is 400iu. Recent medical research indicates that human daily requirements of vitamin D may be up to 10x more than this. If you consider that the skin will naturally produce approximately 10,000iu vitamin D in response to 20–30 minutes summer sun exposure, you can easily see how 400iu might be considered too low!

If you have had a blood test and know your current levels, www.grassrootshealth.net has a fantastic calculator that you can use to determine how much you need to take. You put in your weight, current levels and desired levels and it calculates how many iu you need to get there. You will need to convert your nmol reading to their ng reading (UK to US) – they have a handy serum level converter on the home page too.

Vitamin D doesn't work alone!

Vitamin D has to have help from certain co-factors to work properly in the body. These include the other fat-soluble vitamins K2, E and A as well as minerals such as magnesium, boron, manganese and zinc. So if you start supplementing with vitamin D, make sure you are also getting these co-factors as well or you risk causing more imbalances.

I recommend a good quality multivitamin, plus a vitamin D complete ideally with K2 as a co-factor. See Chapter 11 for more information on supplements.

Please check with your doctor or health practitioner before starting any new supplements, especially if you have a health condition or you are pregnant.

SUMMARY

- Get sun exposure, without sunscreen, for 20 minutes whenever possible (without burning)
- Eat oily fish, egg yolks, and organ meats (e.g. liver) to top up your levels during the winter
- Get tested to know your levels
- Supplement with D3 during the winter months
- Supplement with D3 co-factor vitamins and minerals (vitamins A, E, K, magnesium, zinc, boron)

CHAPTER 8

MINDSET – GET YOUR HEAD SORTED

Now if you're going to do this on your own, there's often something missing. If you don't have this missing piece of the puzzle, your chances of success are limited.

The missing piece is your MINDSET.

Before you change your body, you need to change your mind.

In Chapter 2 we had a look at which of your hormones might be out of balance, where the gap is between where you are now and where you'd like to be, and we looked at your big WHY motivation.

In this chapter we're going to have a closer look at the two major obstacles that might be stopping you achieving results and being the best version of yourself you can be.

Have you got time for this?

The first reason you might have for not taking action is TIME.

'I don't have time to eat healthily'

'I don't have time for exercise'

'I don't have time for relaxation'

If these are some of the things you catch yourself saying, I'd like you to try something.

Instead of 'I don't have time' I want you to say:

'It's not a priority'.

I learnt this little trick years ago, and it has been monumental in changing my frame of mind.

Instead of saying…'I'd love to eat healthier but I just don't have time', it now becomes 'I'd love to eat healthier but "eating healthier isn't a priority for me".'

Suddenly, you realize that your health might not be the priority that you think it is.

There are 168 hours in a week. And we all know that time is our greatest resource. Your priorities, whether you say so or not, are where you choose to spend those hours.

It's amazing how much time you can find when you prioritize the things that are important. Making a commitment to yourself, setting a target date and having something to aim for, that's when you finally make that first step.

If you take a long time either thinking about doing something or even try to go it alone without any support or accountability, life will generally get in the way and before you know it, you are back in your daily routine.

It's so often NOT about what we know – it's about getting it done.

I know this because once my clients start making small achievements, it builds momentum and then when they start losing their excess weight, regaining their energy and feeling balanced, they all say the same thing…

'I should have done this years ago!'

It's not about willpower

The second thing we use as an excuse is willpower, or lack of it.

I'm hoping that if you've got this far, then you're serious and committed to getting your hormones back into balance. But I'm guessing that if you're reading this book you may have tried others before it. If those methods have failed, don't be hard on yourself.

It's so easy to read a book, an article and think, 'Yes, that's what I need to do.' You imagine yourself happier, slimmer, sexier and energetic. You have great intentions to start on Monday; you get the food shopping in and make plans for your meals. The first few days go well, then the weekend comes along and you have a few glasses of wine and polish off the whole box of chocolates. You then think, 'oh well, I've ruined it now, might as well give up!'

I have done this so many times myself. I feel so bad about it afterwards and blame my pathetic willpower. But each time this happens you lose a bit more faith in yourself, and your guilt meter goes up and up. These negative emotions just add to your stress levels and, guess what, your hormones go even more haywire, making you crave more carbs and you pile on even more weight and feel even more exhausted.

STOP!!

You must not blame yourself. It's your hormones that are out of whack, not you! Until you stop beating yourself up, you won't be able to make the changes.

SUMMARY

- Before you can change your body, you need to change your mind
- If you don't have time to be healthy, it might not be your top priority
- It's not about your lack of willpower; it's your hormones that are controlling you!

CHAPTER 9

KEEPING IT GOING

Like I said right at the start, I'm not interested in diets, quick fixes, magic pills or one-off programmes. They are just not going to give you long-term results.

If you follow the principles in the Happy Hormone Code, you will get sustainable benefits. But I know that it's easy to fall off the wagon and slip back to your old ways.

So I'm going to take you through my recommendations for some easy ways to keep it going and make this part of your life forever, not just for the short term.

Get personal!

Sticking to the hormone-friendly food principles that I laid out in Step 1 is a great way to eat FOREVER. The recommended foods are based on a healthy mix of protein, carbs and fats that is designed to keep your weight down, your metabolism firing and energy levels high. It's a preventative strategy for chronic disease too.

The general principles are good ones. They work to lower blood sugar, increase metabolism and improve nutrient stores.

But everyone is different. Every one of us has a unique genetic blueprint and individual biochemistry. While a healthy diet is recommended for everyone, a one-size prescription definitely doesn't fit all.

So it's important to make this personal.

1. Listen to your body
Test yourself – eliminate gluten and dairy from your diet for three to four weeks. If after that you want to test to see if you have an intolerance to either of them, you can do this by bringing them back one at a time and noting your symptoms. Try gluten first – have a decent amount of food containing gluten (like a thick slice of bread/toast or bowl of pasta). Note down any symptoms or reactions (even if it's not gut related, like a headache, for example, or sluggishness or low mood). You may notice obvious bloating or indigestion, or you may just have a low-grade fatigue. But you should notice something if you are sensitive after three to four weeks of going without. Do the same for dairy. Your body's signals should be much clearer now than they used to be. If you do suspect you are sensitive then it's best to avoid it for the long term. Makes sense, right?

2. Take what works, ditch what doesn't
There will be parts of this book that you love (and your body will love too!), and maybe other parts that won't suit you so well. Perhaps you bloat out when you eat grains (even the gluten-free ones). Or you don't digest nuts very well (or you have an allergy). Or you don't react well to eating beans or legumes.

Whatever it is, just design your programme to suit you, and of course your lifestyle. If you manage to get your family eating this way too, that's fantastic – you won't want to go back!

Keep your good habits going. If you lose your sweet tooth (which is very likely), don't start eating sugar again! If you go alcohol free for a few weeks and don't miss it, maybe your body is thanking you. It might be the best thing for you.

3. Keep experimenting – get curious and stay creative
Experiment in the kitchen. Try new smoothies! They are a great way to start your day, avoid the afternoon slump or replace lunch. Whatever you decide, try and do them regularly if you have found a recipe you love. Even if it's just a few times a week.

The 80:20 rule

The 80:20 rule is really important. I don't believe healthy living is sustainable unless you have a break now and then. It certainly works that way for me. I am in no way a saint when it comes to food and drink!

I love my red wine and at the weekends let it go past the recommended daily limit!! Shock horror. But I try to stick to the red stuff, which is healthier than other alcoholic drinks and I do have wine-free days during the week.

I also love chocolate and will indulge in a whole bar if it's left in front of me! It is the dark kind mind you, but still not good in that quantity.

I try to stay gluten free because I know I get bloated when I eat it. But I won't panic if I mistakenly have a bit of wheat or treat myself to the odd slice of chocolate cake.

I try to live by the 80:20 rule. 80% of the time eating heathily, 20% less so. I don't always use my 20% allowance, but I like to know it's there. This rule does several things:

1. **It stops you turning into a freak!** Once you get started on the healthy lifestyle, you can easily get obsessive. They have a name for it now – orthorexia. It can lose you your family and friends and make you go crazy (seriously!).

2. **It allows you to eat away from home.** You can't always stick to the rules when you go out to restaurants, parties or friends' houses. Sometimes you just have to pitch in (unless of course you have food allergies or sensitivities!).

3. **It gives you some room to let go.** Sometimes you just need that piece of chocolate cake, or that freshly baked slice of bread or that super chilled glass of Sauvignon Blanc. Don't deprive yourself if you REALLY want something, just make it a 20% treat and enjoy every last mouthful. Don't you dare feel guilty afterwards though – that will stress your body and undo all the pleasure you just got from the food.

SUMMARY

- Personalize your programme as only you know how!
- Listen to your body
- Be curious and experiment
- Don't obsess or turn into a freak
- Live healthily most of the time
- Be good to yourself

PART 4

BEYOND DIET AND LIFESTYLE

Introduction

Now that you have made positive impacts on the four big influences affecting your hormone health – diet, stress, environment and lifestyle – you should have more control over your hormones, weight, energy, mood and overall health.

If you have had positive results from acting on the advice in this book, are you curious to see how healthy you can actually get? How much more weight you could lose? Or how much more energy you could enjoy? Or even how to adopt the latest anti-ageing techniques that can help prevent the risk of chronic disease?

You may still have some niggling symptoms, OR feel like you have more to achieve (more energy, more weight loss, more hormone balance)?

If you still have some symptoms, you may have something deeper going on. Diet and lifestyle can go a long way, but sometimes you just need a bit more targeted help. Often there's something underlying that is hampering your progress. Common issues are more serious hormone imbalances, digestive issues, toxic overload or nutrient deficiencies.

This section will help you if you want to take any of this further. I explain what tests are available both through your doctor and privately so that you have the tools you need to take more responsibility for your own health. Doctors are extremely busy and don't have as much time as you do to focus on your health! The more informed you are, the better results you are likely to achieve.

I also show you some of my favourite supplements for women over 40. The supplement market is a minefield so I hope this will save you valuable time and money.

And finally some thoughts about hormone replacement therapy, the pros and cons of synthetic vs natural and what choices you have.

CHAPTER 10

GET YOURSELF TESTED

Hormones work to the 'Goldilocks principle' – not too much, not too little, but just right. This is why the 'one size fits all' standard medical approach doesn't always work for everyone, and why if you can afford to invest in more comprehensive tests, you'll get more personalised treatment which can be much more effective.

When we work with clients, we take a full medical history and go through all their symptoms. That usually gives us a good idea about what their hormones are up to. But symptoms are just an indication, and sometimes there are underlying factors that may not be so obvious. That's when testing is so useful for us in clinic.

Testing takes out the guesswork. Even though we're pretty intuitive when it comes to hormones, we like to have the backup of a physical test – because we're not infallible, and we want the absolute best for our clients – so if we know FOR SURE that something isn't where it should be, then we can put a protocol in place that laser targets that specific imbalance – and that helps in three ways:

- The client will get much quicker and more effective results – after all, that's what we're aiming for!
- It helps the client stick to the programme. It's all well and good telling them you have a problem, but seeing it on paper makes it REAL
- It gives us a baseline so we can measure the client's progress from beginning to end

'Normal' or optimal?

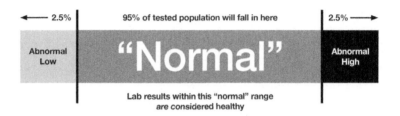

Many clients report that they have had tests done by their doctors and have been told they are 'normal'.

What I often find when I look at the results is that they have fallen into the 'normal' range, however, at the very low end.

If you fall within the normal range, the computer will not flag up your results as needing any action. I hope that most doctors will look through the results anyway and spot any low (but 'normal') readings, but I suspect that many don't get time to do a thorough check.

Unfortunately there's a huge difference between someone with optimal TSH (thyroid stimulating hormone) and someone with a level that is just within range. Or someone with ferritin (iron) at the low end of the range and someone with optimal levels. It will most often show up in their symptoms.

If you ask me, I'd be wanting OPTIMAL levels not 'normal' levels! That's how we work with our clients. Getting them to optimal. It makes a huge difference to their well-being.

The Functional "Optimal" Range

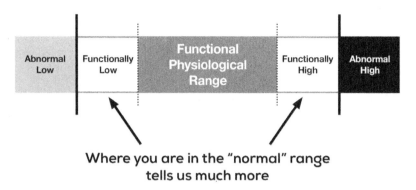

Where you are in the "normal" range
tells us much more

Cortisol testing

As I explained in Chapter 3, chronic stress is at an epidemic level in modern-day society, and this can take a toll on your adrenal glands. A cortisol imbalance over the long term can have serious implications for your health, including cardiovascular, hormones, digestion, neurological and immune function.

Your doctor may test your cortisol levels but it is not a standard test. If your doctor suspects very low or very high levels, he may order a blood test that measures your cortisol levels in the morning. They may be looking for abnormally low levels, which could indicate a serious condition called Addison's disease. They are not looking to measure how well your adrenals are coping over the course of your day. 'Adrenal fatigue' or cortisol imbalance is not a recognized condition in conventional medicine.

Even if you do get your cortisol tested, measuring morning cortisol is not a great way of assessing adrenal health. Your cortisol may be raised if you are rushing to a blood test facility before the school run or work. Measuring cortisol in blood is not the most accurate measure either. And only taking a snapshot of one moment in time is not showing you the pattern of cortisol output during the day.

The alternative? We use a urine test to measure cortisol levels over 4 points in a 24-hour day to check how much cortisol you're producing and what the pattern is. This tells us a huge amount about how your adrenals are coping with any stress you are under – whether that's external stress in your daily life, or internal stress like an underlying infection, hormone imbalance or nutrient deficiency.

It also measures your DHEA, which helps to balance out cortisol, so if you're low (or high) it can indicate adrenal stress.

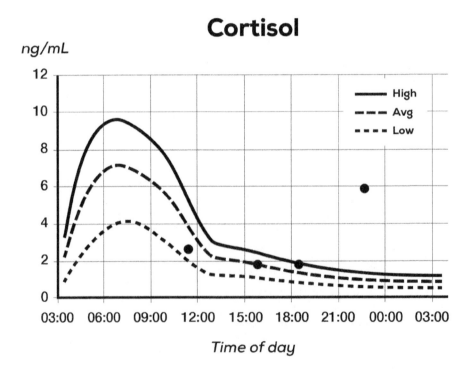

This is a typical adrenal test result. Cortisol should be high in the morning to wake you up, and then taper off during the day with low levels in the evening to prepare for sleep. As you can see, this client's cortisol production was a bit back to front, and she had high levels in the evening preventing her from getting off to sleep at night.

Who might benefit from an adrenal stress test?

Anyone who has the following symptoms:
anxiety, overwhelm, irritability, feeling wired, poor sleep, brain fog, memory loss, digestive issues, frequent colds/infections, PMS, depression, low libido, high blood pressure, palpitations, infertility and belly fat.

Thyroid testing

As you saw in Chapter 3, your thyroid hormone is vital for every cell in the body to make the energy required for it to do its job – whether that's making your heart beat, your muscles work or your brain function properly!

Doctors in general are quite happy to test your thyroid, especially if you have symptoms of fatigue, weight gain, hair loss or have a family history. They will often measure your TSH, T4 and sometimes your thyroid antibodies. These are all important, but they don't always show the whole picture.

Remember the thyroid pathway in Chapter 3? TSH and T4 are just the start of it:

- **TSH** is your thyroid-stimulating hormone – released from the pituitary gland in the brain to tell the thyroid gland how much T4 hormone to make

- **T4** is the inactive hormone that gets converted to T3, your active hormone
- **T3** is the one that does all the work, and this is often not measured
- **RT3** is Reverse T3, produced to inhibit T3 function
- **TPO** (thyroid peroxidase) and **Tg** (thyroglobulin) antibodies – these are the antibodies that target parts of your thyroid gland or receptors

There are three main problems with standard thyroid testing:

1. A very wide reference range
The reference ranges for thyroid hormones are very wide. That means that you could be 'normal' even though you are at the lowest end of the scale. Unless you dip under the threshold you won't get any treatment. This is known as 'subclinical' hypothyroidism and there is much debate about how or even whether it should be treated. Similar to adrenal function, thyroid disease is often only recognized as overt hyperthyroidism and overt hypothyroidism. The thresholds for these diagnoses are:

Hyperthyroid – low TSH (almost undetectable) and high T4

Hypothyroid – high TSH (in the UK typically above 4 or 5mU/L) and/or low T4

If you are producing too much TSH, it indicates that the body doesn't have enough T4 or T3 and is signalling the pituitary to produce more; so more TSH is released. This is a **hypothyroid** condition, and is the most common of the two.

There are many differing views on the lowest reference range for TSH and this is reflected in the variety of lab ranges across the world. Here in the UK, you could have a TSH of just under 5mU/L and be diagnosed 'normal'. However, many health practitioners like to see TSH levels below 2.5 for optimal health, corresponding with published guidelines for pregnant women.

2. It's not the whole picture

The standard initial test for thyroid will sometimes only measure TSH levels. Often T4 is measured though not always in its free form (fT4). It's really important to know your free T4 and free T3 levels but these won't necessarily be measured if your TSH is 'normal'. This testing process only looks at a small part of the HPT axis and doesn't take into account what may be happening further down the chain (e.g. if your T4 is not converting to T3, or you have high antibodies indicating an autoimmune condition).

3. No interest in the cause

If you have low thyroid function, it is vital to know if it is autoimmune related. Around 80% of thyroid disease cases are due to autoimmune Hashimoto's or Graves' disease. Autoimmune thyroid conditions have a different aetiology than other thyroid issues, and so require a different protocol of treatment. Many people are just put on thyroxine, not knowing they have an immune disorder and how to treat it.

If you suspect you may have a thyroid issue, make sure you ask your doctor for all available thyroid measures; TSH, fT4, fT3, and TPO antibodies.

Testing your body temperature at home can be a good initial indication of low thyroid – see Home Thyroid Test in the Resources section. It's sometimes useful to take your results to your doctor if you're trying to get tests done.

The alternative? A full thyroid hormone panel is our standard test for our clients. It includes TSH, fT4, fT3 and TPO antibodies. That way, if there is a problem we can see where in the chain it's likely to be occurring and put in place the right protocol to address it. We will also measure RT3 separately if results come back normal and symptoms persist.

Who might benefit from a full thyroid panel?

Anyone who has the following symptoms:
fatigue, weight gain, anxiety, depression, cold hands/feet, brain fog, memory loss, constipation, PMS, infertility, low libido, hair loss, poor nails, dry skin, joint pain, high cholesterol.

Women over 40 and anyone with a family history of thyroid disease are at a higher risk.

Sex hormone testing

From the age of 35 a woman's sex hormones start to decline (and fluctuate). These are the peri-menopausal years and they can last up to post-menopause (average age 51). Some women sail through this time, but for many it can be a roller coaster. If you have symptoms in your 40s, your doctor may get your FSH (Follicle Stimulating Hormone) and LH (Luteinizing Hormone) levels tested. If these are raised it can indicate that you are in the perimenopause. Not that useful as you probably know that already!

You may also get your oestradiol and sometimes progesterone tested and, if low, HRT (hormone replacement therapy) may be recommended.

Before you opt for HRT, please read Chapter 12 on BHRT (body-identical hormone replacement) so that you can start doing your own research and make an informed decision that's right for you.

Test alternatives? We use in my opinion the best hormone test in the world! It's a dried urine test that not only measures your sex hormone levels but also the metabolites, which gives us a picture of how hormones are actually performing, and crucially how they are being detoxified and eliminated. This is very useful in understanding the behaviour of oestrogen in the body and potential risks of further conditions, including breast and ovarian cancer.

Who might benefit from a sex hormone panel?

Anyone who has the following symptoms:
fatigue, weight gain, anxiety, depression, hot flushes, night sweats, brain fog, memory loss, over-emotional, PMS, heavy/painful periods, breast tenderness, dry skin, vaginal dryness.

In addition, this test can be useful for anyone with a hormone-driven condition, such as PCOS, endometriosis, fibroids and PMS or menstrual issues.

Gut Testing

Stool testing has come a long way in recent years. We use a test that utilizes cutting-edge technology to provide a true DNA-based assessment of your gut microbiome from a single stool sample.

Who might benefit from a gut test?

Anyone with the following symptoms;
IBS, bloating, constipation, diarrhoea, flatulence, indigestion, acid reflux, pain or cramps.

Or other systemic symptoms which may be caused by digestive imbalances such as the following:
migraines, fatigue, brain fog, feeling hungover, depression, anxiety, joint pain, cravings or unexplained weight gain.

Or you have been diagnosed with any of the following:

IBS, Chron's disease, Ulcerative Colitis, Diverticulitis, Colitis or any other inflammatory bowel condition.

Blood tests

Blood testing is most commonly used to detect any health issues relating to blood chemistry, complete blood count, heart, liver, kidney, key nutrients such as vitamin D, B12, ferritin and folate. Also available as standard medical tests are thyroid hormones, as well as key markers for diabetes and inflammation.

There are some limitations however with standard blood testing;

- Reference ranges can be wide so you want to be looking for optimal levels not just 'normal'.
- Some nutrients are not routinely tested such as vitamin D, vitamin B12, iron and folate.
- Thyroid testing is often limited to TSH and T4, not the full pathway.

Private blood testing is an alternative way to get a more comprehensive picture, but you must ensure you get professional help to interpret your results.

If you're interested in discussing testing further please contact us via the website: www.happyhormonesforlife.com/contact

SUMMARY

- Comprehensive testing can often provide the missing piece of the jigsaw.
- Look for optimal not normal when looking at results.
- Useful hormone tests include cortisol, DHEA, a full thyroid panel, vitamin D and all 3 sex hormones.

CHAPTER 11

HOW SUPPLEMENTS CAN HELP

Why do we need to supplement?

Although healthy food always comes first, modern life means that you aren't necessarily getting all the nutrients you need, even if your diet is super healthy.

There are many reasons why:

1. **Nutrient-poor diets** – your diet might be high in refined carbohydrates, sugar, trans-fats and food chemicals, and lacking in nutrient-rich fruit, veg, whole foods and healthy fats.

2. **Soil quality** – today's soils are often depleted of minerals – a study done in 2003 found that compared to the 1930s, the fruit and vegetables we eat contain 20% fewer minerals (zinc and calcium were around 50% lower).

3. **Pesticides** used to grow crops can affect the nutrient content of the food.

4. **Food miles** – long distance transportation of foods depletes nutrient content.

5. **Processing** – the adding of preservatives and additives can decrease nutrient quality.

6. **Stress** – adrenal stress can deplete certain nutrients, leaving us needing additional supplies.

7. **Poor digestion** – ageing, food sensitivities, inflammation and infection can all affect absorption of vital nutrients.

8. **Climate and culture** – it's virtually impossible to get enough vitamin D if you live in a country with very little sunshine through the winter (like the UK) or if you cover up or avoid the sun.

9. **Perimenopause** – as hormones start to decline and fluctuate, we need to ramp up our nutrient intake, and at the same time our absorption capacity can decline.

10. **Medications, smoking, alcohol and caffeine** – can all deplete the body of essential nutrients.

This is why I use supplements, which do exactly as the name implies, they supplement a balanced diet and are not a replacement for it. It can be likened to building a boat with rotten wood and using the best screws that money can buy. It may hold together, but it will leak. Therefore, if you choose poor quality foods, the body will not be working optimally even with the best supplements.

But where do you start? The range of supplements available can be overwhelming, with some brands making ambitious claims. Many of them however contain vitamins and minerals in forms that the body may not be able to absorb very easily (often because they're cheaper). Also, they can contain contaminants, cheap fillers and added sugar or sweeteners. A good quality supplement contains nutrients in the correct balance, and in the best most absorbable form.

As we age, our needs for certain nutrients increase. As women, we also need nutrients for our hormones to work properly.

From my clinical experience, as a general rule these are **my top five** essential supplements for women over 40 (depending on your circumstances):

1. A good quality **multivitamin** – unless you are being tested for every nutrient that you need, this is your basic insurance policy! But I don't recommend any old brand from your supermarket or pharmacy. You must look for good levels of B vitamins and minerals in the right forms, as these are critical in maintaining good hormone function.

2. **Vitamin D3** – most people know that vitamin D is essential for healthy bones, and is therefore important for preventing osteoporosis. However, recent research has suggested that vitamin D can also provide protection from diabetes, high blood pressure, cardiovascular disease, depression, and cancers of the breast, prostate, and colon. Unless you live in year-round sunshine, you will need a vitamin D top-up. And make sure you are also taking its co-factor nutrients (vitamins A, E, K2, magnesium, zinc, boron).

    It's very important to get yourself tested to see where your levels are before supplementing. You can do this through your own doctor or health practitioner, or you can order an inexpensive home test kit from a reputable source. See Chapters 7 and 10 for more details.

3. **Omega 3 fish oil** – the Omega 3 and 6 fats are critical for the structure of your cell membranes, for reducing inflammation and in the prevention of chronic disease (see Chapter 5 for more on fat). Unless you are eating oily fish at least three times a week, you are likely not getting enough Omega 3 fats in the form of EPA and DHA and will need to supplement.

    There is a huge variety of fish oil supplements out there, but many are contaminated with heavy metals or have gone rancid. It's really important to buy a good quality reputable brand, with decent levels of EPA and DHA. For vegetarians or vegans, you can buy non-fish derived Omega 3 supplements.

4. **Magnesium** – this critical mineral is actually responsible for over 300 enzyme reactions and is found in all of your tissues – but mainly in your bones, muscles and brain. You must have it for your cells to make energy, for many different chemical pumps to work, to stabilize membranes and to help muscles relax. And it gets used up really quickly if you're stressed!

There are many different ways of increasing your magnesium:

- Epsom salts – magnesium sulphate salts are great if you don't like taking pills. Put a couple of handfuls in a warm bath and relax for 20 minutes.
- Magnesium oil – you can rub this into your skin.
- Magnesium glycinate or citrate capsules are well-absorbed forms of oral magnesium.

5. **Vitamin C** – this is one vitamin we can't make ourselves (we're in the minority in the animal world here). It's not just for your common cold. It really is vital for your whole immune system. It's antibacterial, antiviral and antifungal, and provides you with vital antioxidant protection against DNA damage and arterial damage. Vitamin C also gets depleted very quickly when there's any stress about, so make sure you are taking more when you're stressed.

You can get vitamin C everywhere. It's normally comes as 'ascorbic acid', but if you have any digestive sensitivity to it you can take it as a mineral ascorbate (e.g. magnesium or calcium ascorbate).

So that's my top five everyday supplements for women over 40. In addition, you may want to look at more specific supplements for certain conditions:

PMS

- Vitamin B6 – can help stimulate progesterone (to balance high oestrogen)
- Magnesium (high dose for pain management) – can help relax uterine muscles
- Vitex agnus-castus – this herb can be useful for increasing progesterone; typically supplement during luteal phase – days 14–28 of cycle
- Fibre – such as psyllium husk can help to eliminate waste oestrogen
- Liver support formula – can help optimize detoxification of excess oestrogen

Hot flushes

- Herbal support including sage, isoflavones, black cohosh, hops, dong quai – can all be helpful
- Adrenal support – many hot flushes are triggered by stress or anxiety (or alcohol!)
- Consider body-identical hormone replacement (see Chapter 12)

Stress

- Magnesium is vital in the production of energy for adrenal function
- B vitamins are needed for hormone production and B5 in particular which helps activate the adrenals
- Vitamin C – used up very quickly by stress hormones

- Herbal adaptogens – such as rhodiola, ashwagandha, holy basil, American ginseng
- Phosphatidylserine – very useful if you have high cortisol
- Liquorice root extract is useful for low cortisol
- Maca powder – this is a Peruvian superfood (available online or in health stores) that can help with stress, energy, and sex drive

Blood sugar balance

- Chromium picolinate can help to control blood sugar and improve the action of insulin
- Cinnamon can help to lower insulin resistance (and improve cholesterol)
- Berberine can help cellular take-up of glucose (therefore improving blood sugar control)
- Adrenal support – cortisol keeps blood sugar high, so reducing stress is vital

You can find links to my favourite brands at www.happyhormonesforlife.com/shop-now.

If you're going it alone, you need to be very careful – the supplement market is a minefield. Just because something is marketed as 'healthy' does not mean it's any good for you! Get advice from someone qualified. You may be doing more harm than good.

The information in this book is for informational purposes only and is not intended as a substitute for medical advice.

You should consult with a doctor or health care professional before taking any new supplements, especially if you have or suspect you have a health condition, are pregnant or you are on medication.

SUMMARY

My top five supplements:

- Multivitamin complex – with good levels of B vitamins and minerals
- Vitamin D3 (with K2) – especially through the winter if you're not getting any sun exposure
- Magnesium
- Fish oil (EPA/DHA)
- Vitamin C

You can find links to my favourite supplement brands here; www.happyhormonesforlife.com/shop-now

CHAPTER 12

HORMONE REPLACEMENT THERAPY – THE LOW-DOWN

Working with women's hormones day in day out, I get asked a lot about HRT. While it's my job to know about treatment options, I am not a medical doctor. I recommend every woman do their own research so they can make an informed decision that's right for them. In this chapter I will summarize my own research on it but I do stress that these are only my opinions and not professional recommendations.

Many women can get relief from menopausal symptoms just by changing their diet and lifestyle, and taking some targeted supplements. However, every woman is unique and while diet and lifestyle can make a huge difference, replacing hormone levels can be a life saver for many women. And vital if you have had an early menopause or a surgically induced menopause (partial or full hysterectomy or oophorectomy).

BENEFITS of hormone replacement

- **Bones** – sex hormones have a vital role to play in bone health. Hormone replacement can help reduce bone loss, and therefore your risk of osteoporosis.
- **Heart** – oestrogen and testosterone can protect the arteries and heart from damage.
- **Skin** – oestrogen reduces collagen loss, therefore helping iron out those wrinkles.
- **Vaginal dryness** – oestrogen can help to keep passageways supple and lubricated.

- **Muscles** – both oestrogen and testosterone help with muscle repair.
- **Brain health, mood and memory** – together with testosterone, oestrogen can improve verbal memory, mood and cognitive function.
- **Stress and sleep** – progesterone is the antidote to stress. It can help to combat the excitatory effects of cortisol and calm the system down.
- **PMS** – using natural progesterone during perimenopause can ease the symptoms of excess oestrogen (including PMS, heavy periods, breast tenderness and fluid retention).
- **Hot flush relief** – oestrogen replacement can help reduce symptoms of hot flushes and night sweats.

The HRT Controversy

So if there are that many benefits, why aren't we all having hormone replacement? There is a lot of controversy in the medical world about how best to restore hormonal balance. And this can be very confusing for women.

The benefits of HRT had been promoted since the 1950s and it was standard practice for women to take it once they reached menopause. However, in 2002, a large study by the Women's Health Initiative (WHI) in the US sent a shock wave when it revealed that HRT (those taking a mix of Premarin and Provera) increased a woman's risk of heart disease, stroke and breast cancer. Many women stopped taking it, and advice was given to those taking it to only take it for a short period of time.

So many women were scared to take, and stay on, HRT for long periods, leaving them facing a tough choice: to risk serious disease, or to suffer menopausal symptoms forever. After the

WHI scare, hormone replacement therapy in women aged 50–59 subsequently dropped by a whopping 79%. A study published in 2013 followed a sample of these women for 10 years, after which they estimated that 50,000 women in this age group may have died prematurely by avoiding oestrogen replacement.

The Different Types Of HRT

Synthetic HRT – Conventional hormone replacement therapy in the form of synthetic hormones used to be the standard medical treatment for most women. These synthetic hormones act in a similar way to your own natural hormones, but they are molecularly different to your own hormones.

We've moved away from the days of being given oestrogen from pregnant horse urine (yes seriously!), but we are still commonly prescribed synthetic hormones in the form of oral oestrogens and progestogens (not progesterone) that are taken orally or in a combined patch.

These synthetic hormones are the ones associated with increased health risks and side effects. However, even these forms of HRT are not as risky as the media would have you believe. Your risk of breast cancer for example is much higher if you're obese or drink too much alcohol.

Body or Bio Identical HRT – Fortunately there are modern forms of HRT that are much safer. More and more doctors are switching to 'body-identical' hormone replacement. The terms Body Identical and Bio Identical are one and the same thing. The NHS doctors know them as Body Identical, so that's what you need to ask for if that's what you want. The hormones used here are still made in the lab, but are chemically identical to your own hormones. They are obtained primarily from plants (soya beans and wild yams), and pharmaceutically transformed to human body-identical hormones. Oestrogen is usually given as a patch (make sure it's oestrogen only), gel or spray. There's only one natural Progesterone (micronized) brand and it is in capsule form.

Bio-identical hormones from private doctors and clinics have been criticized by some medical professionals as unsafe and unproven as the compounding pharmacies that produce them are not widely regulated. However, they have become popular as many GPs are still reluctant to prescribe body-identical HRT, they include testosterone and DHEA (not available currently on the NHS) and they are made to order for your exact dose by the compounding pharmacy.

Is BHRT any safer?

Naturally occurring body-identical hormones are not thought to carry the same risks, as the body treats them in a similar way to your own hormones. They don't have the same side effects either, as your body can metabolize them properly (unlike synthetic hormones).

More studies are needed to ensure that there are no risks to taking body-identical hormones, but so far results look promising.

In a paper published by Kent Holtorf, MD, in 2009, he summarizes the bio-identical debate with these words: 'with respect to the risk of breast cancer, heart disease and stroke, substantial scientific and medical evidence demonstrates that bio-identical hormones are safer and more efficacious forms of HRT, than commonly used synthetic versions.'

A paper published in 2005 took results from 23 years of clinical practice and concluded that bio-identical hormones were safe and effective. A French study looked at over 3000 women using natural progesterone and oestradiol – with no increased health risks.

Another recent study (the EPIC Study) found that a combination of natural oestrogen and progesterone showed evidence of a significant lower risk of breast cancer than other types of HRT.

But hormones are delicately balanced, so even with body-identical hormones, an excess or deficiency in one or more can result in adverse symptoms or increased risk of a hormone-related disease.

Every woman is different. I know women who thrive on HRT, while many who don't want to or can't take hormones, have managed to deal with their symptoms without any prescriptions at all. The most important thing is that you take responsibility for your own health and make sure you're fully informed:

1. Do your own research and always get a second opinion.
2. If your doctor is not helpful, find a new one!
3. Or work with a qualified health professional who can support you and advise you on your options.
4. Get tested – tests can show your hormone levels, how efficiently you are metabolizing and detoxifying your hormones and whether there are any other health risks or genetic factors that could affect your treatment. As we have seen in this book, there are many factors that can upset your hormone balance, and they all need to be considered before embarking on any hormone replacement therapy.

A woman's life expectancy in the 21st century in the western world is now over 80 (according to the World Health Organization). The average age of menopause is 51. That means that we will be living potentially for 30 years in post-menopause so it's important to make sure those years are the best they can be!

SUMMARY

- Hormone replacement has many benefits, including reducing risks of osteoporosis, heart disease and dementia
- HRT is just sex hormone replacement. Diet and lifestyle are still your foundation for all your other hormones
- Modern body-identical HRT is safe and effective
- Do your research and be fully informed to make the choice that's right for you
- Make sure you push for what you need. Many doctors are still to catch up on menopause training.

A FINAL WORD...

So congratulations on coming this far! If you're reading this you're obviously committed to making your life the best it can be at whatever age you happen to be.

We are all 'work in progress' – me included.

I can't live like I used to in my 20s and 30s. I certainly can't pack away the quantities of wine that I used to (never mind the vodka shots and cocktails!) without seriously paying for it in the morning – and that's my liver telling me to change my ways – OK, I'm listening!

I have to exercise smarter and eat so much better just to stay the same weight – no more fad diets for me; they just don't work. I don't restrict calories; I just concentrate on nutrient-rich foods and plenty of healthy fats. If I eat bread and pasta I pay for it by feeling sluggish and bloated – OK I get it!

My knees and hips hurt when I go running – so I now walk more (and have more time to enjoy the scenery!).

I have more lower back issues from sitting a lot – so I have to do more stretching than ever before (I have discovered the joys of yoga!).

And I have to seriously watch my adrenals – so I have started to meditate for 20 minutes every morning (I NEVER thought I could sit still for that long, but I've grown to love my little bit of peace!).

If I don't do all this I know I don't feel great. It's a pretty clear choice.

That's not to say I always make the right one! I'm not perfect – I try to live by the 80:20 rule – 80% healthy (mostly during the week) and 20% a bit more relaxed (mostly the weekends!). It works for me and keeps me sane.

And if you're reading this thinking you're fine – well you may just be one of the lucky ones. I salute (and envy) you! But the majority of women over 40 will have less than optimal energy levels, unwanted weight (especially round the middle), memory or concentration issues, and other symptoms that can indicate hormone imbalances.

And if this is you, I just want you to know that you don't have to put up with it – there is HELP OUT THERE!

If you want to feel good again, it just takes some commitment – either to sorting it out yourself or to getting some help from an expert. Hormone imbalances respond brilliantly to a few tweaks to your diet and lifestyle – you'd be amazed how much!

We all know old habits are very hard to change.

You could walk away from this book with everything you have just learnt, and STILL go straight back to trying the latest fad diet or exercise programme.

I don't want that to happen. My mission in life is to get every woman over 40 back to their best – because as I already told you, it has such a huge ripple effect on everyone around you – it's just too big to not do it.

Changing your thinking around years of the diet trap, to looking after your hormones instead – this is what really works.

At some point you need to put yourself first… And I want that to be NOW.

And hey, if you can get your family living this way too, you'll be giving them the best gift you can.

I really hope you will take on the commitment and prioritize your health NOW. After all, how many lives would be improved if you were at your absolute best?

The rewards are definitely worth it. For me there is no other option.

If you have enjoyed this book, and want help to start your journey to balanced hormones, find out more about all our resources over at www.happyhormonesforlife.com

RESOURCES

To help you put the principles of this book into practice, I have put together some helpful resources for you, including a selection of my favourite hormone-balancing recipes, a guide to eating low GL, my Happy Hormones Plate, the Happy Hormones Manifesto, a helpful home thyroid test and my personal recommendations for websites and further reading.

All of these resources are available to download and print out at www.happyhormonesforlife.com/book

RECODES

Here is a selection of easy and delicious hormone-balancing recipes taken from my 30 Days to Happy Hormones online course. Try them on your family too; they'll be surprised how tasty they are!

Smoothies

Smoothies are so versatile and a great way to balance your blood sugar and pack in the nutrients. If you have a decent blender (mine is a Vitamix, but NutriBullets are a much cheaper option), you can blend pretty much anything into a smooth liquid. Rinse out the blender and you're done – a delicious nutrient-packed drink or meal to go.

Do make sure you are using organic produce for your smoothies; you don't want any pesticides going in there!

Here are three trusted smoothies that I love, to get you started:

Very berry breakfast smoothie (serves 1)

Ingredients
25g gluten-free oats
1 scoop protein powder (organic whey or plant based)
1 scoop superfood greens (I like Life Drink by Terra Nova, but use your favourite)
1 tbsp coconut oil
400ml non-dairy milk of your choice (unsweetened almond, coconut, cashew)
½ banana

1 tbsp mixed seeds
150g frozen berries – blueberries, raspberries, blackberries, strawberries
Handful of ice

Method
Blend all ingredients well and enjoy!

Detox smoothie (serves 1)

Ingredients
1 scoop protein powder (organic whey or plant based)
1 scoop superfood greens (I like Life Drink by Terra Nova, but use your favourite)
5cm piece of cucumber
Handful of lettuce
2cm piece courgette
2cm piece celery
½ apple
½ avocado
Handful of herbs (I like parsley and mint)
Squeeze of lemon juice
400ml unsweetened coconut water
Handful of ice

Method
Blend all ingredients well and enjoy!

Maca chocolate smoothie

Ingredients
1 scoop protein powder (organic whey or plant based)
250ml almond milk (unsweetened)
½ can of coconut milk

1 tbsp maca
1 tbsp raw cacao
½ banana
1 tsp cinnamon
Some ice cubes

Method
Blend all ingredients well and enjoy!

Optional add-ins:
Coconut oil
Olive oil
Flax or hemp oil
Maca powder
Ground flaxseeds
Seeds (raw and unprocessed) – pumpkin seeds, sunflower seeds, chia seeds, hemp seeds, sesame seeds
Cinnamon
Greens – kale, salad leaves, cabbage, chard, etc
Avocado
Herbs – parsley, mint, coriander, basil
Fresh ginger, lemon, lime, orange
Berries
Cucumber, celery, fennel
Nut butters – almond, cashew, hazelnut, macadamia
Vanilla paste
Raw cacao powder or nibs

A note on spinach

I see a lot of green smoothie recipes based on spinach as your main green. While spinach is undoubtedly nutritious and doesn't alter the taste of your smoothie, the issue I have with it is that it contains high amounts of oxalates. Oxalates convert to oxalic acid in your body, and too much can cause calcium oxalate kidney stones (very painful!). A handful of spinach is around 45g, and the recommendation if you are susceptible to oxalates is no more than 30g. Switch to lower oxalate greens such as kale, chard, cabbage, rocket, bok choy or salad leaves for your smoothies and eat your spinach cooked, or raw in small amounts.

Breakfasts

Breakfast is important to fuel you after your overnight fast, and by making it protein/fat based, your blood sugar will be nice and balanced from the start. It will also keep you full til lunchtime.

If you're busy in the morning and don't have much time, then throwing together a smoothie (and taking it with you) is a great option. If you've made a batch of granola then you can have that with full-fat organic milk, a non-dairy milk or natural yoghurt (coconut yoghurt is a great option).

Or you can make a Bircher muesli (see below) the night before and it's ready to go in the morning.

If you have a bit more time or are fairly hungry, you can make eggs pretty quickly.

I love to make pancakes at the weekend, so have included one of my favourite pancake recipes.

Two eggs (serves 1)

Ingredients
2 eggs (fried in coconut oil, poached, boiled or scrambled)
Bacon (organic, free range) or smoked salmon (wild Alaskan)
Assorted veg (e.g. spring onions, greens, spinach, peppers)

Method

Cook eggs however you like them – scrambled, poached, fried in coconut oil.

Grill the bacon and/or fry assorted veg in some coconut oil, or add smoked salmon. Serve with eggs.

Bircher muesli (serves 2)

Ingredients
125g gluten-free oats
480ml almond milk (unsweetened) or any other milk of your choice
1 apple, grated or sliced
½ banana, sliced
Juice of half an orange
Squeeze of lemon
1 tbsp mixed seeds (flax, hemp, sunflower, pumpkin)
1 tbsp chia seeds
1 tsp honey (raw preferably)
1 tsp cinnamon

Method

Mix the oats, milk, cinnamon, lemon and orange juice and leave to soak overnight in the fridge. When you're ready to eat it, add your choice of toppings (e.g. grated apple, banana, honey, seeds).

Paleo banana pancakes (makes 10 small pancakes)

Ingredients
60g almond flour
60g coconut flour
3 eggs
1 ripe mashed banana
1 tsp baking powder
½ tsp salt
1 tsp cinnamon
1 tsp vanilla paste
coconut oil for cooking

Method
Blend all ingredients together to make a batter.

Heat coconut oil in a pan. Add spoonfuls of batter to make small pancakes. Leave to cook on a low heat for a few minutes until firm, then flip and cook the other side.

Top with berries, some raw honey, nuts, seeds, coconut cream or natural yoghurt.

These will keep in the fridge for a few days.

Granola (serves 8–10)

Ingredients
25g gluten-free porridge oats
45g buckwheat or quinoa flakes
50g flaked almonds
50g pecans, roughly chopped
50g walnuts, chopped
75g sunflower seeds
75g pumpkin seeds

2 tbsp flaxseeds
1 tsp cinnamon
4 tbsp melted coconut oil
125ml freshly squeezed orange or apple juice (or coconut water)
1 tbsp raw honey
100g goji berries

Method

Mix all dry ingredients together apart from the goji berries. Mix in melted coconut oil, honey and juice or coconut water. Spread mixture on a greased baking tray and bake in a low oven for 30–40 minutes, stirring half way through. After cooling, add in the berries and store in an airtight container.

Lunches/Dinners

I've included a selection of some of my favourite lunch and dinner recipes. The beauty of these recipes is that they are easy to make and very versatile. You can use dinner leftovers for next day lunch too!

Gem lettuce tuna wraps (serves 1)

A great alternative to your tuna sandwich!

Ingredients
2 gem lettuces
1 tin tuna
2 tbsp organic yoghurt (or coconut yoghurt)
1 tbsp tahini
3 spring onions, chopped small
  red pepper, chopped small
½ avocado, chopped small
Juice of half a lemon
Salt and pepper

Method

Pull apart the gem lettuce 'wraps'. Mix up the tuna with all the other ingredients. Pile into each lettuce wrap.

Creamy coconut lentil soup (serves 4)

Packed with nutrients!

Ingredients
200g red lentils
1 tbsp cider vinegar
1 tbsp coconut oil
600ml chicken stock (or vegetable stock)
400ml coconut milk
1 onion
2 cloves garlic
2½cm fresh ginger
1 tsp turmeric
1 tsp cumin powder
1 organic red pepper
Pinch of chilli flakes
Salt and pepper
Juice of a lemon
Handful of coriander or parsley

Method

Soak lentils in water with cider vinegar for a few hours, then rinse them well.

Fry onion, garlic and ginger in coconut oil until soft. Add red pepper, cumin and turmeric and cook for a few minutes. Add lentils, stock, chilli and coconut milk and simmer for 1 hour, stirring occasionally. Check the lentils are tender, add the seasoning and lemon juice and then serve with a handful of coriander (or parsley).

Sardine pâté (courtesy of Ceri Jones, www.naturalkitchenadventures.com)

Try this even if you're not a fan of sardines – I promise it's delicious and a great way of getting your Omega 3s

Ingredients
1 tin of sardines (in olive oil)
1 clove garlic, minced
2 tbsp natural or coconut yoghurt
Juice of 1 lime
20g fresh coriander
½ tsp sea salt
Good twist black pepper
Pinch of cayenne pepper

Method

Drain the sardines, reserving the oil. Place in the food processor with the rest of the ingredients and blitz to a spreadable consistency, adding a little of the reserved olive oil if necessary. Taste and adjust seasoning if necessary. Transfer to a small pot, cover and refrigerate until ready to eat. Serve with oatcakes or in little gem lettuce boats.

Tomato basil chicken (serves 2)

A staple in our house.

Ingredients
1 tbsp lemon juice
2 tsp rosemary
2 tsp olive oil
2 organic chicken breasts
1 tbsp coconut oil
2 large or 4 medium tomatoes, diced

1 tbsp fresh basil
2 onions, minced
2 tsp balsamic vinegar
Salt and pepper

Method

Combine lemon juice, rosemary, oil, salt and pepper in a medium dish and add chicken. Coat on all sides; cover and refrigerate for ½ to 1 hour. Drain marinade and discard.

Grill chicken for 6–8 minutes on each side.

Heat coconut oil and cook onions until soft. Add tomatoes, basil and balsamic vinegar and heat through. Serve with chicken.

Chilli and garlic prawns (serves 2)

Buttery garlicky prawns, what's not to like?

Ingredients
300g raw king prawns
1 red chilli – deseeded and chopped small
3 cloves garlic, minced
2 tbsp butter (or coconut oil)

Method

Heat up coconut oil or butter in frying pan. Add chilli and prawns. Add the garlic and cook until prawns are pink (don't overcook or they will be chewy).

Eat as they are for a quick lunch or serve with rice noodles, vegetables and brown rice or cauliflower rice.

Vegetable frittata (serves 1)

So quick and versatile – you can add bacon or smoked salmon if you want to jazz it up

Ingredients
2 organic eggs
1 tbsp coconut oil
100g cherry tomatoes, cut in half
2 spring onions
Large handful of spinach
1 tbsp nutritional yeast flakes (or grated cheese)
Handful of basil
Handful of parsley

Method

Whisk the eggs with 2 tbsp of water.

Heat the coconut oil in an ovenproof frying pan with 1 tbsp of water. Add the tomatoes, onions and spinach and cook until spinach begins to wilt. Sprinkle over the herbs. Pour in the eggs, cook lightly then sprinkle on nutritional yeast flakes (or cheese) and transfer to a preheated oven. Bake for 10–12 minutes until well-risen and golden brown. If you don't have an ovenproof frying pan, you can put the pan under a hot grill until the eggs are cooked through and golden brown.

Quinoa tabbouleh with feta (serves 4–6)

A great dish to make and store in the fridge for lunches and side dishes

Ingredients
250g cooked quinoa (or mix of quinoa and lentils)
1 bunch spring onions, chopped

½ red or yellow pepper, chopped
Handful of fresh mint
Handful of chopped parsley
1 garlic clove, chopped
1 fresh red chilli, finely chopped
Small cucumber, chopped
Small punnet cherry tomatoes (or 2 large tomatoes), chopped small
100g feta cheese, cubed
1 tbsp hemp seeds (or other seeds of choice)
Juice of 1 lemon
3 tbsp olive oil
Salt and pepper

Method

Place all ingredients in a mixing bowl and toss together lightly. Chill for 1 hour or more to allow flavours to blend.

Roast cod and lentils (serves 4)

A really tasty way of eating fish

Ingredients
2 tbsp coconut oil, plus extra for greasing
2 tsp mild curry powder
4 x 200g pieces thick cod fillet

For the lentils:
200g puy lentils
2 tbsp coconut oil, melted
2 large garlic cloves, finely chopped
1 medium-hot red chilli, deseeded and finely chopped
½ tsp ground cumin
1 small red onion, finely chopped

1 leek, sliced and chopped
4 tbsp fresh chicken stock
Lemon juice, to taste
3 tbsp chopped fresh coriander

Method

If lentils are not precooked, cook them in a pan of simmering water for 20 minutes, or until tender. After 15 minutes, mix the melted coconut oil for the fish with the curry powder. Brush all over the cod and season.

Bake in the oven for 10–12 minutes.

Drain the lentils. Heat the remaining oil in a clean pan. Add the onions, garlic, chilli and cumin. Once sizzling, stir in the lentils and stock, until warmed through. Add the lemon juice and season to taste. Stir in the coriander.

Spoon onto warmed plates. Place the cod on top.

Thai green chicken curry (serves 2–3)

This one ticks all the boxes for me

Ingredients
1 tbsp coconut oil
2 chicken breasts
1 large onion
2 garlic cloves
2½cm piece ginger
1 red chilli
Packet of Thai green paste
Handful of green beans/sugar snaps
Handful of mushrooms
½ can coconut milk

100ml chicken stock
Handful of coriander, chopped

Method

Heat coconut oil in pan. Add onion and gently fry til soft. Add chopped ginger, chilli and garlic, cook for a minute.

Add mushrooms and cook for a minute or two. Add chicken pieces and brown. Add chicken stock and coconut milk, salt and pepper, stir and leave to simmer for 15 minutes, then add green beans/sugar snaps and cook for another 5 minutes.

Add a sprinkling of coriander and serve in a bowl, with brown rice or quinoa.

Baked sweet potato with hummus (serves 2)

Homemade hummus is the best!

Ingredients
2 sweet potatoes
1 x 400g can chickpeas, rinsed and drained
2 tbsp tahini
1 garlic clove (or 1 tsp garlic powder)
Juice of a lemon
2 tbsp olive oil
Salt and pepper

Method

Roast the sweet potatoes in a tray for 40 minutes.

Meanwhile make the hummus. Mix all ingredients in food processor/blender, adding extra oil according to preferred consistency.

Cut the sweet potatoes lengthways and dollop in the hummus. Serve with salad.

Healthy fried chicken (serves 2)

A great alternative to chicken nuggets for the kids!

Ingredients
2 organic chicken breast pieces, chopped into bite-sized chunks
1 egg, beaten
1 cup coconut or almond flour
1 tbsp coconut oil

Method

Heat up coconut oil in frying pan. Put beaten egg in a wide bowl, coconut or almond flour in another bowl. Dip chicken pieces in egg, then the flour. Repeat one more time.

Fry chicken until golden on both sides.

Serve with green salad, vegetables, brown rice or sautéed greens.

Sautéed greens

Who says greens are tasteless?

Ingredients
Large bunch of greens (e.g. kale, chard, collard greens, cabbage)
2 cloves garlic
1⅕cm of fresh ginger
½ small red chilli, deseeded (optional)
1 tbsp coconut oil
2 tsp sherry or cider vinegar
Salt and pepper

Method

Wash greens and slice thinly. Heat coconut oil in a large frying pan. Add chilli, ginger and garlic. Then add greens and cook until wilted. Add vinegar, salt and pepper and serve.

Home-made chicken stock

A great source of collagen – good for your gut, skin, bones and joints. You can use this stock in soups, sauces and gravies.

Ingredients
Bones from a whole organic chicken (or 2!)
1 bay leaf
2 stalks celery, roughly chopped
1 large onion, peeled and roughly chopped
2 carrots, peeled and roughly chopped
Handful of herbs (optional)
Salt and pepper

Method

Put all the ingredients into a large soup pot, cover with cold water and bring to a boil over high heat. Turn the heat to low and simmer with the lid on for 5–10 hours to really get the juices out of the bones.

Let the stock cool then strain into glass containers (I use old jars) to freeze for up to six months. This is great to do in a slow cooker – you can leave it on low overnight.

Desserts

I love desserts! And I know a lot of women who find it hard to give up a sweet treat for good. The good news is that these recipes are not going to derail your healthy lifestyle, as long as you eat them in moderation of course.

Healthy chocolate mousse (makes 8–10)

You won't believe how good this tastes (hint – you can't taste the avocado!)

Ingredients
1 ripe avocado
1 tbsp raw cacao powder
50g soft pitted dates
1 tbsp raw honey
1 tbsp coconut cream
Juice of a lime

Method

Blend all ingredients together until smooth, adjust sweetness to your taste and pop into fridge for a few hours to firm up.

Coconut mango cream (serves 1)

A delicious tropical treat!

Ingredients
1 small tub of coconut yoghurt (I like Coyo or Coconut Collaborative)
1 tsp vanilla paste
1 mango, peeled and chopped

Method

Whizz up all ingredients in a blender, chill and serve.

Super berry 'cheese' cake

A great dessert to make to impress your friends and family

Ingredients

Base:
320g nuts (almonds, macadamias or hazelnuts)
90g pitted medjool dates

Filling:
300g cashew nuts, soaked in water overnight, then drained
Juice of 1 lemon
3 tbsp maple syrup or coconut nectar
3 tbsp coconut oil, warmed
1 tsp vanilla paste

Top:
90g pitted medjool dates
250g fresh or frozen berries (you can choose raspberries, strawberries, blueberries or a mixture)

Method

Grease a 22cm round tin or dish with butter or coconut oil. Blitz the base ingredients in a food processor until well combined. Press the mixture into the dish and pop in the fridge to set.

For the filling, put all the ingredients plus 100ml of water into a blender and blend until smooth. Pour over the base and put into freezer for a couple of hours to set.

For the topping, put ingredients into a blender and blend until smooth. Pour over the cheesecake and it's ready to serve.

Raw chocolate truffles (makes 8–10)

I'd keep these to yourself!

Ingredients
50g walnuts
50g hemp or chia seeds
100g dates
1 tbsp ground almonds
1 tbsp almond butter
50g cacao powder
1 tbsp maca powder
2 tbsp raw honey
Crushed seeds or coconut for rolling

Method

Mix all ingredients in a food processor until you can mould into ball shapes. Coat each truffle in mixed crushed seeds or desiccated coconut.

Chill in fridge until set.

LOW GL GUIDE

Low Glycaemic Load Guide

You might have heard the terms low GI (Glycaemic Index) and low GL (Glycaemic Load) and wondered what the difference is.

Glycaemic Index indicates how rapidly a carbohydrate is digested and released as glucose (sugar) into the bloodstream. A food with a high GI raises blood sugar more than a food with a medium to low GI. But the Glycaemic Index does not take into account the amount of carbohydrate in a food.

Glycaemic Load is calculated by multiplying the Glycaemic Index of a food by the amount of carbs in a 10-gram portion of the food. This is a much more accurate measure of how much a food will affect your blood sugar.

Glycaemic Load of common foods*

Low (good) = Less than 10, Medium (acceptable) = 11–20, High (avoid/limit) = 21+

Starchy staples: Low-GL alternatives

	Low GL	High GL
Bread	Wholegrain 100% (7), rye (10), sourdough (8), soya and linseed (5), barley and sunflower (6), seeded breads (6) and wholewheat pitta breads (8)	White bread (11), bagel (24), French baguette (10), rice cakes (17), white pitta (10)

---

* Adapted from International Tables of Glycemic Index and Glycemic Load Values, *Diabetes* (2008)

	Low GL	High GL
Cereal	Whole oats (11), oatmeal (9), no added sugar muesli (8)	Rice-based cereals (21), bran flakes (13), wheat biscuits (14), cornflakes (23)
Pasta	Rice noodles (15)	Spaghetti (27)
Rice	Brown rice (16), quinoa (13)	White rice (25), sticky white rice (24)
Potatoes	Sweet potatoes (11)	Baked white potatoes (33), French fries (21), mashed potato (26)

Low GL seasonal fruit and vegetables

	Fruits	Vegetables
Spring	Rhubarb, grapes, limes, passion fruit, lemons, grapefruit, avocados	Leeks, cabbage, watercress, new potatoes, spinach, aubergines, radishes, rocket, spring greens
Summer	Strawberries, raspberries, blueberries, redcurrants, blackcurrants, cherries, nectarines, melons	Asparagus, baby carrots, fresh peas, tomatoes, runner beans, lettuce, cucumber, courgettes, peppers, mangetout
Autumn	Blackberries, apples, pears, gooseberries, damsons, plums, elderberries, greengages	Pumpkin, onions, fennel, wild mushrooms, squash, turnips, red cabbage, celeriac, swede
Winter	Satsumas, clementines, cranberries, mandarins, tangerines, pears, pomegranates	Brussels sprouts, chicory, cauliflower, kale, celery, mushrooms, purple sprouting broccoli

THE HAPPY HORMONES PLATE

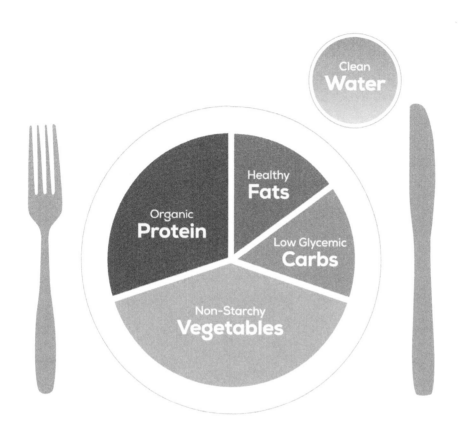

Clean **Water**

Healthy **Fats**

Organic **Protein**

Low Glycemic **Carbs**

Non-Starchy **Vegetables**

THE **HAPPY HORMONES** PLATE

30%	15%	40%	15%
Protein	**Healthy Fats**	**Vegetables**	**Carbs**
ANIMAL	• Organic dairy	• Leafy greens	• Low sugar fruit
• Meat (organic)	• Avocado	• Cabbage	(apples, berries)
• Eggs (organic)	• Olive oil	• Broccoli	• Beans
• Fish (wild caught,	• Coconut oil	• Cauliflower	• Legumes
not farmed)	• Cold pressed	• Carrots	• Sweet potato
	plant oils	• Beets	• Gluten free grains
VEGAN	• Coconut milk	• Courgette	• Quinoa
• Beans	• Almond milk	• Aubergine	• Brown/wild rice
• Nuts, seeds	• Nuts	• Onion	• Gluten free pasta
• Legumes	• Seeds	• Garlic	• Noodles
• Soy (natto, miso,	• Bone Stock	• Cucumber	(buckwheat, rice)
tempeh)		• Asparagus	
• Seaweed		• Salad leaves	

Based on all my studies and clinical experience, I've designed my ideal plate for hormone balance. There's no counting calories or weighing food. For me it's more important to look at maximizing your hormone-boosting nutrients. For this to happen we need the right proportions of protein, fat and carbs.

This plate supports your **Feisty 4** hormones, the ones that control your metabolism, mood, cycle and weight – **cortisol, insulin, thyroid** and **oestrogen**. By reducing food stressors, balancing blood sugar and providing all the essential nutrients for your hormone production, you've got a fighting chance of keeping them balanced and working for you, not against you.

It's also a really healthy way for everyone to eat, so try it out on your family too.

HOME THYROID TEST

While I would always recommend thorough thyroid hormone testing with your doctor or with a qualified health practitioner, this is a useful home test that you can do on yourself to see if you may have a thyroid issue.

The Barnes Basal Test for thyroid function

The Broda Barnes temperature test measures morning basal temperature and can be a possible indicator of deficient thyroid.

1. Keep a thermometer by your bedside at night.
2. When you wake up in the morning, put the thermometer under your armpit for 10 minutes and keep still.
3. Note the temperature after 10 minutes.
4. Repeat for seven mornings.

Pre-menopausal women should start the test on day two of their menstrual cycle. Post-menopausal women and men can start the test on any day.

The normal range for underarm morning temperature is between **36.6°C** (97.8 F) and **36.8°C** (98.2 F). If the recorded temperature is consistently below these levels, a more comprehensive blood test for thyroid is recommended (even if you have been told your initial results are 'normal').

Body temperature is affected by many factors, so this test alone should not be used as a diagnosis.

Day	Temperature
Day 1	
Day 2	
Day 3	
Day 4	
Day 5	
Day 6	
Day 7	

THE HAPPY HORMONES MANIFESTO

HAPPY HORMONES
—— MANIFESTO ——

EAT a rainbow. Love your cruciferous. **real food.** Think protein. Sugar is sneaky. **dark chocolate.** Smile. No guilt.

ENJOY fat. Cook from scratch. **ORGANIC** is best.

Make **green** smoothies. Drink **good** coffee. Stay hydrated.

GREEN and leafy. **COCONUT** is king.

Don't graze. **Fast** overnight.

Fermented foods. **FLAXSEEDS.**

CHILL OUT. RELAX. BREATHE DEEPLY. SIT QUIETLY. SLEEP DEEPLY.

Don't be a stress junkie. **BE PRESENT.**

Get some **SUN.** Be in nature. Touch the **EARTH.**

Laugh. **SEE FRIENDS.** Be grateful. **BALANCE.**

Love your liver. No BPA. **Detox** your world. Essential **oils.**

WALK DAILY. Sit less. **MOVE.** Dance. **STRETCH.**

Chew slowly. Be **MINDFUL.**

DON'T GIVE UP. BE GOOD TO YOURSELF.

www.happyhormonesforlife.com

REFERENCES

Perimenopause

Arpels, J.C. (1996) The female brain hypoestrogenic continuum from the premenstrual syndrome to menopause. A hypothesis and review of supporting data. *J Reprod Med*, 41(9):633–639.

Barth, C. et al. (2015) Sex hormones affect neurotransmitters and shape the adult female brain during hormonal transition periods. *Front Neurosci*, 9:37.

Burger, H.G., Hale, G.E., Dennerstein, L., Robertson, D.M. (2008) Cycle and hormone changes during perimenopause: the key role of ovarian function. *Menopause*,15:603–612.

Davis, S.R. et al. (2012) Understanding weight gain at menopause. Writing Group of the International Menopause Society for World Menopause Day 2012. *Climacteric*, 15(5):419–429.

Greenblum, C.A. et al. (2013) Midlife women: symptoms associated with menopausal transition and early postmenopause and quality of life. *Menopause*, 20(1):22–27.

Hays, B. (2010) Female Hormones: The Dance of the Hormones, Part 1. In Jones, D., ed. *Textbook of Functional Medicine.* Institute of Functional Medicine.

Mitchell, E.S. and Woods, N.F. (2010) Pain symptoms during the menopausal transition and early postmenopause. *Climacteric*, 13(5):467–478.

Nappi, R.E. and Lachowsky, M. (2009) Menopause and sexuality: prevalence of symptoms and impact on quality of life. *Maturitas*, 63(2):138–141.

Prior, J.C. (1998) Perimenopause: the complex endocrinology of the menopausal transition. *Endocr Rev*, 19(4):397–428.

Cortisol and stress

Akerstedt, T. (2006) Psychosocial stress and impaired sleep. *Scand J Work Environ Health*, 32(6):493–501.

Arnett, J.L. et al. (1986) Loss of libido due to stress. *Medical Aspects of Human Sexuality*, 20(1).

Bland, J. (2002) *Nutritional Endocrinology – Breakthrough Approaches for Improving Adrenal and Thyroid Function 2002 syllabus*. pp.82–117, pp.165–167.

Bauld, R. and Brown R.F. (2009) Stress, psychological distress, psychosocial factors, menopause symptoms and physical health in women. *Maturitas*, 62(2):160–165.

Brotto, L.A. and Basson, R. (2014) Group mindfulness-based therapy significantly improves sexual desire in women. *Behav Res Ther*, 57:43–54.

Carlson, L et al. (2004) Mindfulness-based stress reduction in relation to quality of life, mood, symptoms of stress and levels of cortisol, dehydroepiandrosterone sulfate (DHEAS) and melatonin in breast and prostate cancer outpatients. *Psychoneuroendocrinology*, 29(4):448–474.

Charmandari, E. et al. (2005) Endocrinology of the stress response. *Rev Physiol*, 7:259–284.

Chevalier, G. et al. (2012) Earthing: Health Implications of Reconnecting the Human Body to the Earth's Surface Electrons. *J Environ Public Health*, 291541. [Online].

Daubenmier, J. et al. (2011) Mindfulness Intervention for Stress Eating to Reduce Cortisol and Abdominal Fat among Overweight and Obese Women: An Exploratory Randomized Controlled Study. *Journal of Obesity*.

Epel, E. et al. (2000) Stress and body shape: stress-induced cortisol secretion is consistently greater among women with central fat. *Psychosomatic Medicine* 62.

Guilliams, T.G. and Edwards, L. (2013) Chronic Stress and the HPA Axis: Clinical Assessment and Therapeutic Considerations. *The Standard*, 9(2):623–632.

Heitkemper, M. (1996) Increased urine catecholamines and cortisol in women with irritable bowel syndrome. *Am J Gastroenterol*, 91(5):906–913.

McEwen, B.S. and Sapolsky, R.M. (1995) Stress and cognitive function. *Curr Opin Neurobiol*, 5(2):205–216.

Moore, A. and Malinowski, P. (2009) Meditation, mindfulness and cognitive flexibility. *Conscious Cogn*, 18(1):176–186.

Kaliman, P. et al. (2014) Rapid changes in histone deacetylases and inflammatory gene expression in expert meditators. *Psychoneuroendocrinology*, 40:96–107.

Katterman, S.N. et al. (2014) Mindfulness meditation as an intervention for binge eating, emotional eating, and weight loss: A systematic review. *Eat Behav*, 15(2):197–204.

Rakowski, R. (2002) *New Strategies for Improving Adrenal and Thyroid Function 2002 syllabus*.

Segerstrom, S.C. and Miller, G.E. (2004) Psychological stress and the human immune system: a meta-analytic study of 30 years of inquiry. *Psychological Bulletin*, 130(4):601–630.

Thirthalli, J. et al. (2013) Cortisol and antidepressant effects of yoga. *Indian Journal of Psychiatry, 55:S405<N>S408.*

Van Eck, M. et al. (1996) The effects of perceived stress, traits, mood states, and stressful daily events on salivary cortisol. *Psychosom Med*, 58(5):447–458.

Wilson, J.L. (2014) Clinical perspective on stress, cortisol and adrenal fatigue. *Advances in Integrative Medicine* 1(2):93–96.

Winbush, N.Y. et al. (2007) The effects of mindfulness-based stress reduction on sleep disturbance: a systematic review. *Explore* (NY), 3(6):585–591.

Zellner, D.A. et al. (2006) Food selection changes under stress. *Physiol Behav*, 87(4):789–793. Epub 2006 6 Mar.

Sleep

Briffa, Dr J. (2012) Can lack of sleep contribute to obesity? [Online]; http://www.drbriffa.com/2012/02/10/can-lack-of-sleep-contribute-to-obesity/

Kravitz, H.M. et al. (2008) Sleep disturbance during the menopausal transition in a multi-ethnic community sample of women. *Sleep*, 31(7):979–990.

Knutson, K., Spiegel, K., Penev, P., Van Cauter, E. (2007). The Metabolic Consequences of Sleep Deprivation. *Sleep Med Rev*, 11(3):163–178.

Lulu Xie et al. (2013) Sleep Drives Metabolite Clearance from the Adult Brain. *Science*, 342(6156):373–377.

Laugsand, L.E., Vatten, L.J. Platou, C. and Janszky, I. (2011) Insomnia and the Risk of Acute Myocardial Infarction: A Population Study. *Circulation*, 124:2073–2081.

Obal, F. and Krueger, J.M. (2001) *Hormones, Cytokines and Sleep.*

Reiter, R. (1994) Melatonin suppression by static and extremely low frequency electromagnetic fields: relationship to the reported increased incidence of cancer. *Rev Environ Health,* 10(3–4):171–186.

Schernhammer, E.S. and Schulmeister, K. (2004) Melatonin and cancer risk: does light at night compromise physiologic cancer protection by lowering serum melatonin levels? *Br J Cancer,* 90(5):941–943.

Schmid, S.M. (2008) A single night of sleep deprivation increases ghrelin levels and feelings of hunger in normal-weight healthy men. *J Sleep Res,* 17(3):331–334.

Spiegel, K. et al. (2005) Sleep loss: a novel risk factor for insulin resistance and Type 2 diabetes. *Journal of Applied Physiology,* 99(5):2008–2019.

Spiegel, K., Tasali, E., Penev, P., and Van Cauter, E. (2004) Brief Communication: Sleep Curtailment in Healthy Young Men Is Associated with Decreased Leptin Levels, Elevated Ghrelin Levels, and Increased Hunger and Appetite. *Ann Intern Med,* 141:846–850.

Taheri, S., Lin, L., Austin, D. et al. (2004) Short sleep duration is associated with reduced leptin, elevated ghrelin, and increased body mass index. *PLoS Med,* 1(3):e62.

Insulin and blood sugar control

Arcidiacono, B. et al. (2012) Insulin resistance and cancer risk: an overview of the pathogenetic mechanisms. *Exp Diabetes Res.*

Johnson, R. J. et al. (2007) Potential role of sugar (fructose) in the epidemic of hypertension, obesity and the metabolic syndrome, diabetes, kidney disease, and cardiovascular disease. *American Journal of Clinical Nutrition.*

Lakhan, S.E. and Kirchgessner, A. (2013) The emerging role of dietary fructose in obesity and cognitive decline. *Nutr J*, 12:114.

Liu, H. and Heaney, A.P. (2011) Refined fructose and cancer. *Expert Opinions on Therapeutic Targets.*

Ludwig, D.S. (2002) The glycemic index: physiological mechanisms relating to obesity, diabetes and cardiovascular disease. *JAMA*, 287:2414–2423.

Rada, P. et al. (2005) Daily bingeing on sugar repeatedly releases dopamine in the accumbens shell. *Neuroscience*, 134(3):737–744.

Schmidt, J. et al. (2011) Reproductive hormone levels and anthropometry in postmenopausal women with PCOS: A 21 year follow up study. *J Clin Endocrinol Metab*, 96(7).

Schwingshackl, L. and Hoffmann, G. (2013) Long-term effects of low glycemic index/load vs. high glycemic index/load diets on parameters of obesity and obesity-associated risks: a systematic review and meta-analysis. *Nutr Metab Cardiovasc Dis*, 23(8):699–706.

Shiloah, E. et al. (2003) Effect of acute psychotic stress in nondiabetic subjects on beta-cell function and insulin sensitivity. *Diabetes Care*, 26(5):1462–1467.

Thomas, D.E. (2007) Low glycaemic index or low glycaemic load diets for overweight and obesity. *Cochrane Database Syst Rev*, 3:CD005105.

Turner, R. et al. (2013) Individuals with Alzheimer's disease exhibit a high prevalence of undiagnosed impaired glucose tolerance and type 2 diabetes mellitus. *Alzheimer's & Dementia*.

Thyroid

Anderson, P. (2015) Hashimoto's Disease: The Underactive Thyroid Disease. *MSN Student Scholarship*. Paper 121.

Brent, G.A. (2010) Environmental exposures and autoimmune thyroid disease. *Thyroid*, 20(7):755–761.

Hak, A.E. et al. (2000) Subclinical hypothyroidism is an independent risk factor for atherosclerosis and myocardial infarction in elderly women. *Ann Intern Med*, 132(4):270–278.

Helmreich, D.L. et al. (2005) Relation between the hypothalamic-pituitary-thyroid (HPT) axis and the hypothalamic-pituitary-adrenal (HPA) axis during repeated stress. *Neuroendocrinology*, 81(3):183–192. Epub 2005 11 Jul.

Kirkegaard, C. and Faber, J. (1998) The role of thyroid hormones in depression. *European Journal of Endocrinology*, 138:1–9.

Knudsen, N. et al. (2002) Risk factors for goiter and thyroid nodules. *Thyroid*, 12(10):879–888.

Luboshitzky, R., Aviv, A., Herer, P. and Lavie, L. (2002) Risk factors for cardiovascular disease in women with subclinical hypothyroidism. *Thyroid*, 12:421–425.

Maes, M. et al. (1997) Components of biological variation, including seasonality, in blood concentrations of TSH, TT3, FT4, PRL, cortisol and testosterone in healthy volunteers. *Clin Endocrinol* (Oxf), 46(5):587–598.

Metso, S. et al. (2012) Gluten-free diet and autoimmune thyroiditis in patients with celiac disease. *Scandinavian Journal of Gastroenterology*, 47.

Nicolle, L. and Beirne, A.W. (2010) *Biochemical Imbalances in Disease*. London: Singing Dragon, p. 187.

Pizzorno, L. and Ferril, F. (2005) Thyroid. In D.S. Jones and S. Quinn (eds) *Textbook of Functional Medicine*. WA: Gig Harbour.

Uzunlugu, M. et al. (2007) Prevalence of Subclinical Hypothyroidism in Patients with Metabolic Syndrome. *Endocrine Journal*, 54(1):71–76.

Oestrogen

Adlercreutz, H. and Mazur, W. (1997) Phyto-oestrogens and Western diseases. *Ann Med*, 29: 95–120 (Medline).

Barth, C. et al. (2015) Sex hormones affect neurotransmitters and shape the adult female brain during hormonal transition periods. *Front Neurosci*, 9:37.

Behl, C., Skutella, T., Lezoualch, F. et al. (1997) Neuroprotection against oxidative stress by estrogens: structure–activity relationship. *Mol Pharmacol*, 51:535–541.

Borrelli, F. and Ernst, E. (2010) Alternative and complementary therapies for the menopause. *Maturitas*, 66:333–343.

Engler-Chiurazzi, E.B. et al. (2016) Estrogens as neuroprotectants: Estrogenic actions in the context of cognitive aging and brain injury. *Prog Neurobiol*, Feb. 15.

Eisenberg, V.H. et al. (2012) Is there an association between autoimmunity and endometriosis? *Autoimmun Rev*, 11(11):806–814.

Gorbach, S.L. and Goldin, B.R. (1987) Diet and the excretion and enterohepatic cycling of estrogens. *Prev Med*, 16(4):525–531.

Graham, J.D. and Clarke, C.L. (1997) Physiological action of progesterone in target tissues. *Endocr Rev*, 18(4):502–519.

Hajirahimkhan, A., Dietz, B.M. and Bolton, J.L. (2013) Botanical Modulation of Menopausal Symptoms: Mechanisms of Action? *Planta Med*, 79:538–553.

Lokuge S. et al. (2011) Depression in women: windows of vulnerability and new insights into the link between estrogen and serotonin. *Journal of Clinical Psychiatry*, 72(11):e1563-9.

Nelson, L.R. and Bulun, S.E. (2001) Estrogen production and action. *J Am Acad Dermatol*, 45(3 Suppl):S116–124.

Rose, D.P. et al. (1991) High-fiber diet reduces serum estrogen concentrations in premenopausal women. *Am J Clin Nutr*, 54(3):520–525.

Shanafelt, T.D., Barton, D.L., Adjei, A.A. and Loprinzi, C.L. (2002) Pathophysiology and treatment of hot flashes. *Mayo Clin Proc*, (11):1207–1218.

Zava, D.T. et al. (1998) Estrogen and progestin bioactivity of foods, herbs, and spices. *Proceedings of the Society for Experimental Biology and Medicine*, 217(3):369–378.

Food and nutrients

Adlercreutz, H. et al. (1993) Inhibition of human aromatase by mammalian lignans and isoflavonoid phytoestrogens. *J Steroid Biochem Mol Biol*, 44(2):147–153.

Amagase, H. and Nance, D.M. (2008) A randomized, double-blind, placebo-controlled, clinical study of the general effects of a standardized Lycium barbarum (Goji) Juice, GoChi. *J Altern Complement Med*, 14(4):403–412.

Atkinson, F.S. et al. (2008) International Tables of Glycemic Index and Glycemic Load Values. *Diabetes Care*, 31: 2281–2283.

Auborn, K.J. et al. (2003) Indole-3-carbinol is a negative regulator of estrogen. *Journal of Nutrition*, 133(7 Suppl):2470S-2475S.

Balick, M.J. and Lee, R. (2002) Maca: from traditional food crop to energy and libido stimulant. *Altern Ther Health Med*, 8(2):96–98.

Barr, S.B. and Wright, J.C. (2010) Postprandial energy expenditure in whole-food and processed-food meals: implications for daily energy expenditure. *Food Nutr Res*, 2:54.

Boirie, Y, et al. (1997) Slow and fast dietary proteins differently modulated postprandial protein accretion. *Proc Natl Acad Sci U S A*, 94(26):14930–14935.

Bolin Qin et al. (2010) Cinnamon: Potential Role in the Prevention of Insulin Resistance, Metabolic Syndrome, and Type 2 Diabetes. *J Diabetes Sci Technol*, 4(3):685–693.

Carlsson, S. et al. (2005) Alcohol consumption and type 2 diabetes: Meta-analysis of epidemiological studies indicates a U-shaped relationship. *Diabetologia*, 48(6):1051–1054.

Dabas, D. et al. (2013) Avocado (Persea americana) seed as a source of bioactive phytochemicals. *Curr Pharm Des*, 19(34):6133–6140.

Dennis, E.A. et al. (2010) Water consumption increases weight loss during a hypocaloric diet intervention in middle-aged and older adults. *Obesity*, 18(2):300–307.

Freedman, N.D, Park, Y., Abnet, C.C. et al. (2012) Association of coffee drinking with total and cause-specific mortality. *N Engl J Med*, 366:1891–1904.

Genta, S. et al. (2009) Yacon syrup: beneficial effects on obesity and insulin resistance in humans. *Clin Nutr*, 28(2):182–187.

Hassan, S.T.S. et al. (2016) Antimicrobial, antiparasitic and anticancer properties of Hibiscus sabdariffa (L.) and its phytochemicals: in vitro and in vivo studies. *Ceska Slov Farm*, 65(1):10–14.

Hatori, M. et al. (2012) Time-restricted feeding without reducing caloric intake prevents metabolic diseases in mice fed a high-fat diet. *Cell Metab*, 15(6):848–860.

Higdon, J.V. et al. (2007) Cruciferous Vegetables and Human Cancer Risk: Epidemiologic Evidence and Mechanistic Basis. *Pharmacol Res*, 55(3):224–236.

Hyman, M. (2012) *The Blood Sugar Solution*. [Kindle version] London: Hodder & Stoughton.

Joy, J.M. et al. (2013) The effects of 8 weeks of whey or rice protein supplementation on body composition and exercise performance. *Nutr J*, 12:86.

Kohmani, E.F. (1939) Oxalic acid in foods and its behaviour and fate in the diet. *Journal of Nutrition*, 18(3):233–246.

Lakhan, S.E. et al. (2009) Inflammatory mechanisms in ischemic stroke: therapeutic approaches. *Journal of Translational Medicine*, 7:97.

Lieberman, S. and Bruning, N. (2007) *The Real Vitamin & Mineral Book*. New York: Avery.

Lindahl, G. et al. (2011) Tamoxifen, flaxseed, and the lignan enterolactone increase stroma- and cancer cell-derived IL-1Ra and decrease tumour angiogenesis in estrogen-dependent breast cancer. *Cancer Res*, 71(1):51–60.

Liska, D. (2004) *Clinical Nutrition: A Functional Approach.* Washington: Institute for Functional Medicine.

Loenneke, J.P. et al. (2012) Quality protein intake is inversely related with abdominal fat. *Nutr Metab*, 9(1):5.

Martin, F.P. et al. (2009) Metabolic effects of dark chocolate consumption on energy, gut microbiota, and stress-related metabolism in free-living subjects. *J Proteome Res*, 8(12):5568–5579.

Panahi, Y. et al. (2015) Chlorella vulgaris: A Multifunctional Dietary Supplement with Diverse Medicinal Properties. *Curr Pharm Des*, 22(2):164–173.

Park, Y.M. et al. (2015) A high-protein breakfast induces greater insulin and glucose-dependent insulinotropic peptide responses to a subsequent lunch meal in individuals with type 2 diabetes. *J Nutr*, 145(3):452–458.

Pelucchi, C. et al. (2011) Alcohol consumption and cancer risk. *Nutr Cancer*, 63(7):983–990.

Prasad, K. (2001) Secoisolariciresinol diglucoside from flaxseed delays the development of type 2 diabetes in Zucker rat. *J Lab Clin Med*, 138:32–39.

Pruthi, S. et al. (2007) Pilot evaluation of flaxseed for the management of hot flashes. *J Soc Integr Oncol*.

Qinghua Wu et al. (2016) The antioxidant, immunomodulatory, and anti-inflammatory activities of Spirulina: an overview. *Arch Toxicol*, 90(8):1817–1840.

Rohrmann, S. et al. (2007) Intake of heterocyclic aromatic amines from meat in the European Prospective Investigation into Cancer and Nutrition (EPIC) – Heidelberg cohort. *British Journal of Nutrition*, 98(6):1112–1115.

Schauss, A.G. et al. (2006) Antioxidant capacity and other bioactivities of the freeze-dried Amazonian palm berry, Euterpe oleraceae mart (acai). *J Agric Food Chem*, 54(22):8604–8610.

Shearer, J. and Swithers, S.E. (2016) Artificial sweeteners and metabolic dysregulation: Lessons learned from agriculture and the laboratory. *Rev Endocr Metab Disord*, 17(2):179–186.

Srednicka-Tober, D. et al. (2016) Composition differences between organic and conventional meat: a systematic literature review and meta-analysis. *Br J Nutr*, 115(6):994–1011.

Steinbrecher, A. and Linseisen, J. (2009) Dietary Intake of Individual Glucosinolates in Participants of the EPIC-Heidelberg Cohort Study. *Ann Nutr Metab*, 54:87–96.

Stohs, S.J. and Hartman, M.J. (2015) Review of the Safety and Efficacy of Moringa oleifera. *Phytother Res*, (6):796–804.

Swithers, S.E. (2013) Artificial sweeteners produce the counterintuitive effect of inducing metabolic derangements. *Trends Endocrinol Metab*, (9):431–441.

Wanders, A.J. et al. (2011) Effects of dietary fibre on subjective appetite, energy intake and body weight: a systematic review of randomized controlled trials. *Obes Rev*, 12(9):724–739.

Westerterp-Plantenga, M.S. et al. (2012) Dietary protein – its role in satiety, energetics, weight loss and health. *Br J Nutr*, 108 (Suppl 2):S105–112.

Zhang, W. et al. (2008) Dietary flaxseed lignan extract lowers plasma cholesterol and glucose concentrations in hypercholesterolaemic subjects. *British Journal of Nutrition*, 99:1301–1309.

Zhu, H. et al. (2009) Cruciferous dithiolethione-mediated coordinated induction of total cellular and mitochondrial antioxidants and phase 2 enzymes in human primary cardiomyocytes: cytoprotection against oxidative/electrophilic stress and doxorubicin toxicity. *Exp Biol Med* (Maywood), 234(4):418–429.

Fat

Assunção, M.L. et al. (2009) Effects of dietary coconut oil on the biochemical and anthropometric profiles of women presenting abdominal obesity. *Lipids*, 44(7):593–601.

Brinton, E.A. et al. (1990) A low-fat diet decreases high density lipoprotein (HDL) cholesterol levels by decreasing HDL apolipoprotein transport rates. *J Clin Invest*, 85(1):144–151.

Gillman, M.W. et al. (1997) Margarine intake and subsequent coronary heart disease in men. *Epidemiology*, 8(2):144–149.

Harcombe, Z. et al. (2015) Evidence from randomised controlled trials did not support the introduction of dietary fat guidelines in 1977 and 1983: a systematic review and meta-analysis. *Open Heart*, 2: doi:10.1136/openhrt-2014-000196.

Kavanagh, K. et al. (2007) Trans fat diet induces abdominal obesity and changes in insulin sensitivity in monkeys. *Obesity* (Silver Spring), 15(7):1675–1684.

Mozaffarian, D. and Willet, W.C. (2009) Health effects of trans-fatty acids: experimental and observational evidence. *Eur J Clin Nutr*, 63 (Suppl 2):S5-21. doi: 10.1038/sj.ejcn.1602973.

O'Keefe, S. et al. (1994) Levels of Trans Geometrical Isomers of Essential Fatty Acids in Some Unhydrogenated US Vegetable Oils. *Journal of Food Lipids*, 1:165–176.

Parks, E.J. et al. (1999) Effects of a low-fat, high-carbohydrate diet on VLDL-triglyceride assembly, production, and clearance. *J Clin Invest*, 104(8):1087–1096.

St-Onge, M.P. and Jones, P.J. (2002) Physiological effects of medium-chain triglycerides: potential agents in the prevention of obesity. *J Nutr*, 132(3):329–332.

St-Onge, M.P. et al. (2003) Medium-chain triglycerides increase energy expenditure and decrease adiposity in overweight men. *Obes Res*, 11(3):395–340.

Siri-Tarino, P.W. et al. (2009) Meta-analysis of prospective cohort studies evaluating the association of saturated fat with cardiovascular disease. *Am J Clin Nutr*, 91(3):535–546.

Wansink, B. and Chandon, P. (2006). Can 'Low-Fat' Nutrition Labels Lead to Obesity? *Journal of Marketing Research*, 43(4):605–617.

The Weston A. Price Foundation, *The Oiling of America*.

Yancy Jr., W.S. et al. (2004) A low-carbohydrate, ketogenic diet versus a low-fat diet to treat obesity and hyperlipidemia: a randomized, controlled trial. *Ann Intern Med*, 140(10):769–777.

Environment and toxins

Anetor, J.I. et al. (2008) High cadmium / zinc ratio in cigarette smokers: potential implications as a biomarker of risk of prostate cancer. *Niger J Physiol Sci*, 23(1–2):41–49.

Byford, J.R. et al. (2002). Oestrogenic activity of parabens in MCF7 human breast cancer cells. *Journal of Steroid Biochemistry & Molecular Biology*, 80:49–60.

Calafat, A., Ye, X., Wong, L.Y., Reidy. J. and Needham, L. (2008) Exposure of the U.S Population to Bisphenol A and 4-tertiary-Octylphenol: 2003–2004. *Environmental Science and Technology*, 116:39–44.

Carwile, J., Luu, H., Bassett, L. et al. (2009) Polycarbonate bottle use and urinary bisphenol A concentrations. *Environ Health Perspectives*, 117(9):1368–1372.

Crinnion, W.J. (2010) Toxic effects of the easily avoidable phthalates and parabens. *Altern Med Rev*, 15(3):190–196.

Davis, D.L., Bradlow, H.L. et al. (1993) Medical hypothesis: xenoestrogens as preventable causes of breast cancer. *Environ Health Perspect*, 101(5):372–377.

Environmental Working Group, Skin Deep. Butylated Hydroxyanisole, [Online]: http://www.ewg.org/skindeep/ingredient/700740/BHA/. Accessed 20 June 2013.

Goldman, L.R. (2007) Managing pesticide chronic health risks: U.S. policies. *J Agromedicine*, 12(1): 67–75.

Kapoor, D. and Jones, T.H. (2005) Smoking and hormones in health and endocrine disorders. *Eur J Endocrinol*, 152(4):491–499.

Lee, D.H. et al. (2011) Low Dose Organochlorine Pesticides and Polychlorinated Biphenyls Predict Obesity, Dyslipidemia, and Insulin Resistance among People Free of Diabetes. *PLoS One*, 6(1):e15977.

Lin, C.Y. et al. (2009) Association Among Serum Perfluoroalkyl Chemicals, Glucose Homeostasis, and Metabolic Syndrome in Adolescents and Adults. *Diabetes Care*, 32(4):702-707.

Lind, P.M., Zethelius, B. and Lind, L. (2012) Circulating levels of phthalate metabolites are associated with prevalent diabetes in the elderly. *Diabetes Care*, 35(7):1519–1524.

Marsee, K. et al. (2007). Estimated Daily Phthalate Exposures in a Population of Mothers of Male Infants Exhibiting Reduced Anogenital Distance. *Environ Health Perspect*, 114(6): 805–809.

Nielsen, S.E. et al. (2013) Hormonal contraception use alters stress responses and emotional memory. *Biol Psychol*, 92:257–266.

Pelton, R. et al. (1999) *Drug-Induced Nutrient Depletion Handbook*, Lexicomp Clinical Reference Library – See more at [Online]: http://drhoffman.com/article/drugs-that-steal-2/#sthash.4Lef6Pgz.dpuf Accessed 12 November 2016.

Ropero, A.B. et al. (2008) Bisphenol–A disruption of the endocrine pancreas and blood glucose homeostasis. *Int J Androl*, 31(2):194–200.

Schectman, G. et al. (1989) The influence of smoking on vitamin C status in adults. *Am J Public Health*, 79(2):158–162.

Schlumpf, M. et al. (2004) Endocrine activity and developmental toxicity of cosmetic UV filters – an update. *Toxicology*, 205(1):113–122.

Strunecka, A. et al. (2007) Fluoride Interactions: From Molecules to Disease. *Current Signal Transduction Therapy*, 2(3):190–213.

Teitelbaum, S.L. et al. (2012). Associations between phthalate metabolite urinary concentrations and body size measures in New York City children. *Environ Res*, 112:186–193.

US Environmental Protection Agency. TSCA Chemical Substances inventory; [Online]; http://www.epa.gov/oppt/existingchemicals/pubs/tscainventory/basic.html Accessed 12 November 2016.

Viñas, R. and Watson, C.S. (2013) Mixtures of xenoestrogens disrupt estradiol-induced non-genomic signaling and downstream functions in pituitary cells. *Environ Health*, 12:26.

WHO 2012 State of the Science of Endocrine Disrupting Chemicals. [Online]; http://apps.who.int/iris/bitstream/10665/78102/1/WHO_HSE_PHE_IHE_2013.1_eng.pdf Accessed 12 November 2016.

Wong, P.K. et al. (2007) The effects of smoking on bone health. *Clin Sci* (Lond), 113(5):233–241.

Gut and liver

Blaser, M. (2011) Antibiotic overuse: Stop the killing of beneficial bacteria. *Nature*, 476(7361):393–394.

Budak, N.H. et al. (2014) Functional properties of vinegar. *Journal of Food Science*, 79(5).

Clemente, J. et al. (2012) The impact of the gut microbiota on human health: an integrative view. *Cell*, 148.

Dalen, J. et al. (2010) Pilot Study: Mindful Eating and Living (MEAL): weight, eating behavior, and psychological outcomes associated with a mindfulness-based intervention for people with obesity. *Complement Ther Med*, 18(6):260–264.

David, L.A. et al. (2014) Diet rapidly and reproducibly alters the human gut microbiome, *Nature*, 505:559–563.

Gallant, L. (2014) The gut microbiome and the brain. *J Med Food*, 17(12):1261–1272.

Gill, H.S. and Guarner, F. (2004) Review; Probiotics and human health: a clinical perspective. *Postgrad Med J*, 80:516–526. doi:10.1136/pgmj.2003.008664.

Heitkemper, M.M. and Chang, L. (2009) Do fluctuations in ovarian hormones affect gastrointestinal symptoms in women with irritable bowel syndrome? *Gend Med*, 6(Suppl 2):152–167.

Itan, Y. et al. (2010) A Worldwide Correlation of Lactase Persistence Phenotype and Genotypes. *BMC Evolutionary Biology*, 9 February.

Konturek, P.C. et al. (2011) Stress and the gut: pathophysiology, clinical consequences, diagnostic approach and treatment options. *J Physiol Pharmacol*, 62(6):591–599.

Petsiou, E.I. et al. (2014) Effect and mechanisms of action of vinegar on glucose metabolism, lipid profile, and body weight. *Nutr Rev*, 72(10):651–661.

Ritchie, M.L. and Romanuk, T.N. (2012) A meta-analysis of probiotic efficacy for gastrointestinal diseases. *PLoS One*, 7(4):e34938.

Sender, R. et al. (2016) Revised estimates for the number of human and bacteria cells in the body. BioRxiv.org.

Timmerman, G. and Brown, A. (2012). The Effect of a Mindful Restaurant Eating Intervention on Weight Management in Women. *Journal of Nutrition Education and Behavior*, 44(1):22–28.

Visser, J. et al. (2009) Tight junctions, intestinal permeability, and autoimmunity: celiac disease and type 1 diabetes paradigms. *Ann N Y Acad Sci*, 1165:195–205. doi: 10.1111/j.1749-6632.2009.04037.x.

Xuan, C. et al. (2014) Microbial Dysbiosis Is Associated with Human Breast Cancer. *PLoS One*, 9(1):e83744.

Gluten

Biesiekierski, J.R. et al. (2011) Gluten causes gastrointestinal symptoms in subjects without celiac disease: a double-blind randomized placebo-controlled trial. *Am J Gastroenterol*, 106(3):508–14; quiz 515.

Catassi, C. et al. (2013) Non-Celiac Gluten Sensitivity: The New Frontier of Gluten Related Disorders. *Nutrients*, 5:3839–3853.

Ouaka-Kchaou, A. et al. (2008) Autoimmune Diseases in Coeliac Disease: Effect of Gluten Exposure. *Therap Adv Gastroenterol*, 1(3):169–172.

Tovoli, F. et al. (2015) Clinical and diagnostic aspects of gluten related disorders. *World J Clin Cases*, 3(3):275–284.

Vazquez-Roque, M.I. et al. (2013) A controlled trial of gluten-free diet in patients with irritable bowel syndrome-diarrhea: effects on bowel frequency and intestinal function. *Gastroenterology*, 144(5):903-911.e3.

Exercise

Beddhu, S. et al. (2015) Light-intensity physical activities and mortality in the United States general population and CKD subpopulation. *Clin J Am Soc Nephrol*, 10(7):1145–1153.

Borghouts, L.B. and Keizer, H.A. (2000) Exercise and insulin sensitivity: a review. *Int J Sports Med*, 21(1):1–12.

Fowke, Jay H. (2014) A New Instrument to Comprehensively Assess Sedentary Behaviors. Vanderbilt University Medical. http://grantome.com/grant/NIH/R01-NR011477-05.

Harner, H.M. et al. (2012) Physical activity, stress reduction, and mood: insight into immunological mechanisms. *Methods in Molecular Biology*, 934:89–1002.

Jayabharathi, B. and Judie, A. (2014) Complementary health approach to quality of life in menopausal women: a community-based interventional study. *Clin Interv Aging*, 9:1913–1921.

Kossman, D.A. et al. (1985) Exercise lowers estrogen and progesterone levels in premenopausal women at high risk of breast cancer. *J Appl Physiol*, 111(6):1687–1693.

Lees, S.J. and Booth, F.W. (2004) Sedentary death syndrome. *Can J Appl Physiol*, 29(4):447–460; discussion 444–446.

Moore, S.C. et al. (2012) Leisure time physical activity of moderate to vigorous intensity and mortality: a large pooled cohort analysis. *PLoS Med*, 9(11).

Nevill, M.E., Holmyard, D.J., Hall, G.M. et al. (1996) Growth hormone responses to treadmill sprinting in sprint- and endurance-trained athletes. *European Journal of Applied Physiology and Occupational Physiology*, 72(5-6):460–467.

Salmon, P. (2001) Effects of physical exercise on anxiety, depression, and sensitivity to stress: a unifying theory. *Clin Psychol Rev*, 21(1):33–61.

Sim, A.Y. et al. (2013) High-intensity intermittent exercise attenuates ad-libitum energy intake. *International Journal of Obesity*, Advance online publication 9 July.

Trapp, E.G., Chisholm, D.J., Freund, J. and Boutcher, S.H. (2008) The effects of high-intensity intermittent exercise training on fat loss and fasting insulin levels of young women. *International Journal of Obesity*, 32(4):684–691.

Weuve, J. et al. (2004) Physical activity, including walking, and cognitive function in older women. *JAMA*, 292(12):1454–1461.

Dieting and calorie model

Gornall, J. and Villani, R.G. (1996) Short-term changes in body composition and metabolism with severe dieting and resistance exercise. *Int J Sport Nutr*, 6(3):285–294.

Redman, L.M. et al. (2009) Metabolic and behavioral compensations in response to caloric restriction: implications for the maintenance of weight loss. *PLoS One*, 4(2):e4377.

Tomiyama, A.J. et al. (2010) Low calorie dieting increases cortisol. *Psychosom Med*, 72(4):357–364.

Testing

Baisier, W.V., Hertoghe, J. and Eckhaut, W. (2000) Thyroid Insufficiency: Is TSH the only Diagnostic Tool? *J Nutrit Environ Med*, 10:105–113.

Edelman, A. et al. (2007). A comparison of blood spot vs. plasma analysis of gonadotropin and ovarian steroid hormone levels in reproductive-age women. *Fertility and Sterility*, 88(5):1404–1407.

Inder, W.J. et al. (2012) Measurement of salivary cortisol in 2012 – laboratory techniques and clinical indications. *Clin Endocrinol (Oxf)*, 77(5):645–651.

Meier, C., Trittiback, P., Fuflielmetti, M., Staub, J. and Muller, B. (2003) Serum Thyroid Stimulating Hormone in Assessment of Severity of Tissue Hypothyroidism in Patients with Overt Primary Thyroid Failure: Cross Sectional Survey. *BMJ*, 326(7384):311–312.

Ramakrishnan, L. (2008) Analysis of the Use of Dried Blood Spot Measurements in Disease Screening. *Journal of Diabetes Science and Technology*, 2(2):242–243.

Stagnaro-Green, A. et al. (2011) Guidelines of the American Thyroid Association for the Diagnosis and Management of Thyroid Disease During Pregnancy and Postpartum. *Thyroid*, 21(10): 1081–1125.

Zava, D. et al. (2006) Filter paper dried blood spot assay of insulin measurement. *American Diabetes Association 66th Scientific Sessions*, Washington DC.

Supplements

Anderson, R. et al. (2015) Cinnamon extract lowers glucose, insulin and cholesterol in people with elevated serum glucose. *J Tradit Complement Med*, 6(4):332–336.

A scientific review: the role of chromium in insulin resistance. (2004) *Diabetes Education*, Suppl 2–14.

Barański, M. et al. (2014) Higher antioxidant and lower cadmium concentrations and lower incidence of pesticide residues in organically grown crops: a systematic literature review and meta-analyses. *Br J Nutr,* 112(5):794–811.

Filaretov, A.A. et al. (1986) Effect of adaptogens on the activity of the pituitary-adrenocortical system in rats. *Bull Exp Biol Med,* 101:573–574.

Gröber, U. et al. (2015) Magnesium in Prevention and Therapy. *Nutrients,* 7(9):8199–8226.

Head, K.A. and Kelly, G.S. (2009) Nutrients and botanicals for treatment of stress: adrenal fatigue, neurotransmitter imbalance, anxiety, and restless sleep. *Altern Med Rev,* 14(2):114–140.

Jianghua, L. et al. (2001) Evaluation of Estrogenic Activity of Plant Extracts for the Potential Treatment of Menopausal Symptoms. *J Agric Food Chem,* 49(5):2472–2479.

Johnson, S. (2001) The multifaceted and widespread pathology of magnesium deficiency. *Med Hypotheses,* 56(2):163–170.

Kimura, K. et al. (2007) L-Theanine reduces psychological and physiological stress responses. *Biol Psychol,* 74(1):39–45. Epub 2006 22 Aug.

Mills, S. and Bone, K. (2000). *Principles and Practice of Phytotherapy.* London: Churchill Livingstone.

Monteleone, P. et al. (1990) Effects of phosphatidylserine on the neuroendocrine response to physical stress in humans. *Neuroendocrinology,* 52(3):243–248.

Noreen, E.E. et al. (2010) Effects of supplemental fish oil on resting metabolic rate, body composition and salivary cortisol in healthy adults. *J Int Soc Sports Nutr,* 7:31.

Padayatty, S.J., Katz, A. and Wang, Y. et al. (2003) Vitamin C as an antioxidant: evaluation of its role in disease prevention. *J Am Coll Nutr*, 22(1):18–35.

Panossian, A. and Wikman, G. (2009) Evidence-based efficacy of adaptogens in fatigue, and molecular mechanisms related to their stress-protective activity. *Current Clinical Pharmacology*, 4(3):198–219.

Simopoulos, A.P. and De Meester, F. (2008) A Balanced Omega-6/Omega-3 Fatty Acid Ration, Cholesterol and Coronary Heart Disease. *World Review of Nutrition and Dietetics* Vol. 100, Karger Publications.

Wang, Y. et al. (2013). Effects of vitamin C and vitamin D administration on mood and distress in acutely hospitalized patients. *Am J Clin Nutr*, 98(3):705<N>711.

White, P.J. and Broadley, M.R. (2005) Historical variation in the mineral composition of edible horticultural products. *J Hort Sci Biotechnol*, 80:660–667.

Yin, J. et al. (2008) Efficacy of Berberine in Patients with Type 2 Diabetes. *Metabolism*, 57(5):712–717.

HRT and BHRT

Beral, V. (2003) Million Women Study Collaborators. Breast cancer and hormone-replacement therapy in the Million Women Study. *Lancet*, 362(9382):419–427.

Chen, W., Manson, J., Hankinson, S. et al. (2006) Unopposed estrogen therapy and the risk of invasive breast cancer. *Arch Intern Med*, 166:1027–1032.

Cordina-Duverger, E. et al. (2013) Risk of breast cancer by type of menopausal hormone therapy: a case-control study among post-menopausal women in France. *PLoS One*, 8(11):e78016.

Cowan, L.D. et al. (1981) Breast cancer incidence in women with a history of progesterone deficiency. *Am J Epidemiol*, 114:209–221.

De Lignières, B. et al. (2002) Combined hormone replacement therapy and risk of breast cancer in a French cohort study of 3175 women. *Climacteric*, 5:332–340.

Formby, B. and Wiley, T.S. (1998) Progesterone inhibits growth and induces apoptosis in breast cancer cells: inverse effects on Bcl-2 and p53. *Ann Clin Lab Sci*, 28:360–369.

Holtorf, K. (2009) The bioidentical hormone debate: are bioidentical hormones (estradiol, estriol, and progesterone) safer or more efficacious than commonly used synthetic versions in hormone replacement therapy? *Postgrad Med*, 121(1):73–85.

Rossouw, J.E., Anderson, G.L., Prentice, R.L. et al. (2002) Risks and benefits of estrogen plus progestin in healthy postmenopausal women. *JAMA*, 288(3):321–333.

Sarrel, P.M. et al. (2013) The mortality toll of estrogen avoidance: an analysis of excess deaths among hysterectomized women aged 50 to 59 years. *Am J Public Health*, 103(9):1583–8.

Wright, J. V. (2005) Bio-Identical Steroid Hormone Replacement: Selected Observations from 23 Years of Clinical and Laboratory Practice. *Annals of the New York Academy of Sciences*, 1057:506–524. doi: 10.1196/annals.1356.039.

Vitamin D

Gillie, O. (ed.) Sunlight, Vitamin D & Health (2005) A report of a conference held at the House of Commons in November

2005, organised by the Health Research Forum. Available as a free download from http://www.healthresearchforum.org.uk Accessed 12 November 2016.

Holick, M.F. (2007) Vitamin D deficiency. *New England Journal of Medicine*, 357(3):266–281.

Mohammed Husein Mackawy, A. et al. (2013) Vitamin D Deficiency and Its Association with Thyroid Disease. *International Journal of Health Science* (Qassim), 7(3):267–275.

ScienceDaily (2007) Vitamin D Backed For Cancer Prevention In Two New Studies – 8 February. [Online]; www.sciencedaily.com. Accessed 12 November 2016.

Whitton, C. et al. (2011) National Diet and Nutrition Survey: UK food consumption and nutrient intakes from the first year of the rolling programme and comparisons with previous surveys. *British Journal of Nutrition*, 106(12):1899–1914.

INDEX

Printed in Great Britain
by Amazon

80955961R00188